Nursing Care in the ICU

Nursing Care in the ICU

Guest Editor
Christina Alexopoulou

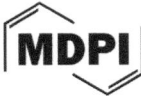

Basel • Beijing • Wuhan • Barcelona • Belgrade • Novi Sad • Cluj • Manchester

Guest Editor
Christina Alexopoulou
ICU Medical School
Democritus University of Thrace
Alexandroupolis
Greece

Editorial Office
MDPI AG
Grosspeteranlage 5
4052 Basel, Switzerland

This is a reprint of the Special Issue, published open access by the journal *Healthcare* (ISSN 2227-9032), freely accessible at: www.mdpi.com/journal/healthcare/special_issues/JK73RF34UY.

For citation purposes, cite each article independently as indicated on the article page online and using the guide below:

Lastname, A.A.; Lastname, B.B. Article Title. *Journal Name* **Year**, *Volume Number*, Page Range.

ISBN 978-3-7258-3144-9 (Hbk)
ISBN 978-3-7258-3143-2 (PDF)
https://doi.org/10.3390/books978-3-7258-3143-2

© 2025 by the authors. Articles in this book are Open Access and distributed under the Creative Commons Attribution (CC BY) license. The book as a whole is distributed by MDPI under the terms and conditions of the Creative Commons Attribution-NonCommercial-NoDerivs (CC BY-NC-ND) license (https://creativecommons.org/licenses/by-nc-nd/4.0/).

Contents

About the Editor vii

Preface ix

Athanasios Theofanopoulos, Athanasia Proklou, Marianna Miliaraki, Ioannis Konstantinou, Konstantinos Ntotsikas and Nikolaos Moustakis et al.
Post-Traumatic Cerebral Venous Sinus Thrombosis (PtCVST) Resulting in Increased Intracranial Pressure during Early Post-Traumatic Brain Injury Period: Case Report and Narrative Literature Review
Reprinted from: *Healthcare* 2024, 12, 1743, https://doi.org/10.3390/healthcare12171743 1

Dragana Simin, Vladimir Dolinaj, Branislava Brestovački Svitlica, Jasmina Grujić, Dragana Živković and Dragana Milutinović
Blood Transfusion Procedure: Assessment of Serbian Intensive Care Nurses' Knowledge
Reprinted from: *Healthcare* 2024, 12, 720, https://doi.org/10.3390/healthcare12070720 10

Varvara Pakou, Dimitrios Tsartsalis, Georgios Papathanakos, Elena Dragioti, Mary Gouva and Vasilios Koulouras
Personality Traits, Burnout, and Psychopathology in Healthcare Professionals in Intensive Care Units—A Moderated Analysis
Reprinted from: *Healthcare* 2024, 12, 587, https://doi.org/10.3390/healthcare12050587 23

Christina Alexopoulou, Athanasia Proklou, Sofia Kokkini, Maria Raissaki, Ioannis Konstantinou and Eumorfia Kondili
A Fatal Case of Presumptive Diagnosis of Leptospirosis Involving the Central Nervous System
Reprinted from: *Healthcare* 2024, 12, 568, https://doi.org/10.3390/healthcare12050568 41

Jéssica Moura Gabirro Fernando, Margarida Maria Gaio Marçal, Óscar Ramos Ferreira, Cleoneide Oliveira, Larissa Pedreira and Cristina Lavareda Baixinho
Nursing Interventions for Client and Family Training in the Proper Use of Noninvasive Ventilation in the Transition from Hospital to Community: A Scoping Review
Reprinted from: *Healthcare* 2024, 12, 545, https://doi.org/10.3390/healthcare12050545 52

Ru-Yu Lien, Chien-Ying Wang, Shih-Hsin Hung, Shu-Fen Lu, Wen-Ju Yang and Shu-I Chin et al.
Reduction in the Incidence Density of Pressure Injuries in Intensive Care Units after Advance Preventive Protocols
Reprinted from: *Healthcare* 2023, 11, 2116, https://doi.org/10.3390/healthcare11152116 65

Silmara Meneguin, Camila Fernandes Pollo, Murillo Fernando Jolo, Maria Marcia Pereira Sartori, José Fausto de Morais and Cesar de Oliveira
Impact of Care Interventions on the Survival of Patients with Cardiac Chest Pain
Reprinted from: *Healthcare* 2023, 11, 1734, https://doi.org/10.3390/healthcare11121734 76

Konstantinos Giakoumidakis, Athina Patelarou, Anastasia A. Chatziefstratiou, Michail Zografakis-Sfakianakis, Nikolaos V. Fotos and Evridiki Patelarou
Development and Validation of the CVP Score: A Cross-Sectional Study in Greece
Reprinted from: *Healthcare* 2023, 11, 1543, https://doi.org/10.3390/healthcare11111543 87

Konstantina Avgeri, Epaminondas Zakynthinos, Vasiliki Tsolaki, Markos Sgantzos, George Fotakopoulos and Demosthenes Makris
Quality of Life and Family Support in Critically Ill Patients following ICU Discharge
Reprinted from: *Healthcare* 2023, 11, 1106, https://doi.org/10.3390/healthcare11081106 97

Paraskevi Stamou, Dimitrios Tsartsalis, Georgios Papathanakos, Elena Dragioti, Mary Gouva and Vasilios Koulouras
Agreement between Family Members and the Physician's View in the ICU Environment: Personal Experience as a Factor Influencing Attitudes towards Corresponding Hypothetical Situations
Reprinted from: *Healthcare* **2023**, *11*, 345, https://doi.org/10.3390/healthcare11030345 . . . . . . **108**

Mohammed Saeed Aljohani
Competency in ECG Interpretation and Arrhythmias Management among Critical Care Nurses in Saudi Arabia: A Cross Sectional Study
Reprinted from: *Healthcare* **2022**, *10*, 2576, https://doi.org/10.3390/healthcare10122576 . . . . . **120**

About the Editor

Christina Alexopoulou

Dr. Christina Alexopoulou is an associate professor of intensive care medicine at the Medical School of Democritus University of Thrace and an ICU consultant at the University General Hospital of Alexandroupolis in Greece.

She graduated in 1993, and she obtained her Ph.D., "Angiogenic Growth Factors in Respiratory Muscles in Adult Patients with Increased Respiratory Load", in 2005 from Medical School, University of Crete, Greece. She also obtained the postgraduate course in "Organization and Management of Health Services", National and Kapodistrian University of Athens, School of Economics.

She worked as a visiting doctor and research fellow at the following institutions:
- Heart and Lung Institute, Imperial College, Royal Brompton and Haerfield Hospital, London, UK.
- Department of Pulmonary, Critical Care, and Sleep Medicine, University of Manitoba, Health Sciences Center, Winnipeg, Manitoba, Canada.
- Intensive Care Unit at Guy's and St. Thomas' NHS, London, UK.

Her research interests include sleep in ICU, nursing in ICU, the physiology of the respiratory system, and mechanical ventilation.

She is the author of articles published in peer-reviewed scientific journals with high impact factors, conference abstracts, and she is the author of several book chapters.

She is a member of the European Society of Intensive Care Medicine, Hellenic Thoracic Society, Hellenic Society of Critical Care, European Sleep Research Society, European Respiratory Society, and a board member of the Hellenic Society of Hypnology.

Preface

The ICU environment is challenging for both patients and staff. The management of critically ill patients is extremely demanding, and the workload and knowledge level required of staff are high. ICU nurses are responsible for the care and treatment of patients in an unstable and/or critical clinical state, assessment of therapies, and the performance of high-intensity interventions. ICU nursing practice includes crucial clinical decisions based on the best available scientific evidence, clinical experience, and patient preferences. ICU nurses carry out specific, autonomous, or complementary interventions of a technical–scientific, managerial, relational, and educational nature; plan healthcare assistance through scientifically validated tools; and identify, analyze, calculate, and treat risks related to care provision by systematically evaluating healthcare outcomes. This reprint consists of eleven chapters, including eight research reports, one review, and two case reports, and is dedicated to the valuable, hardworking, and respected ICU nursing staff.

Christina Alexopoulou
Guest Editor

Case Report

Post-Traumatic Cerebral Venous Sinus Thrombosis (PtCVST) Resulting in Increased Intracranial Pressure during Early Post-Traumatic Brain Injury Period: Case Report and Narrative Literature Review

Athanasios Theofanopoulos [1], Athanasia Proklou [2], Marianna Miliaraki [3,*], Ioannis Konstantinou [2], Konstantinos Ntotsikas [1], Nikolaos Moustakis [1], Sofia Lazarioti [1], Eleftherios Papadakis [2], George Kypraios [4], Georgios Angelidis [4], Georgia Vaki [4], Eumorfia Kondili [2] and Christos Tsitsipanis [1]

1. Neurosurgery Department, University Hospital of Heraklion, School of Medicine, University of Crete, 71003 Heraklion, Crete, Greece; moustakisnik00@gmail.com (N.M.); xtsitsipanis@gmail.com (C.T.)
2. Intensive Care Unit, University Hospital of Heraklion, School of Medicine, University of Crete, 71003 Heraklion, Crete, Greece; proklath@gmail.com (A.P.); kondylie@uoc.gr (E.K.)
3. Pediatric Intensive Care Unit, University Hospital of Heraklion, School of Medicine, University of Crete, 71003 Heraklion, Crete, Greece
4. School of Medicine, University of Crete, 71003 Heraklion, Crete, Greece
* Correspondence: med1p1130027@med.uoc.gr; Tel.: +30-2810392119

Abstract: Post-traumatic cerebral venous sinus thrombosis (ptCVST) often remains underdiagnosed due to the non-specific nature of clinical signs, commonly mimicking severe traumatic brain injury (TBI) manifestations. Early recognition of this rare and potentially life-threatening complication is crucial for the effective management of severe TBI patients in Intensive Care. The present study reports the case of a 66-year-old male who was transferred to the emergency department due to moderate TBI. Initial emergency brain computed tomography (CT) scans revealed certain traumatic lesions, not necessitating any urgent neurosurgical intervention. During his stay in an Intensive Care Unit (ICU), multiple transient episodes of intracranial pressure (ICP) values were managed conservatively, and through placement of an external ventricular drain. Following a series of CT scans, there was a continuous improvement of the initial traumatic hemorrhagic findings despite his worsening clinical condition. This paradox raised suspicion for ptCVST, and a brain CT venography (CTV) was carried out, which showed venous sinus thrombosis close to a concomitant skull fracture. Therapeutic anticoagulant treatment was administered. The patient was discharged with an excellent neurological status. To date, there are no clearly defined guidelines for medical and/or surgical management of patients presenting with ptCVST. Therapy is mainly based on intracranial hypertension control and the maintenance of normal cerebral perfusion pressure (CCP) in the ICU. The mismatch between clinical and imaging findings in patients with TBI and certain risk factors raises the suspicion of ptCVST.

Keywords: traumatic brain injury; cerebral venous thrombosis; post-traumatic; intracranial hypertension; clinical and imaging mismatch

1. Introduction

Post-traumatic cerebral venous sinus thrombosis (ptCVST) often remains underdiagnosed due to its non-specific nature of clinical signs, commonly mimicking severe traumatic brain injury (TBI) manifestations [1,2]. Cerebral venous sinus thrombosis (CVST), whether traumatic or not, constitutes a rare pathological entity, referring to dural venous sinuses clotting and leading to an impaired venous outflow [3,4]. Most reported rates for CVST range from 3–5 per million, while ptCVST is generally reported in 7–35% of TBI cases [1,5]. In ptCVST, trauma-induced venous drainage impairment results in elevated intracranial pressure (ICP) due to cerebral edema, venous infarctions, intraparenchymal hemorrhage, or reduced cerebrospinal fluid reabsorption [6,7]. Among the reported risk factors, the presence of skull fractures, particularly those located close to dural venous sinuses or the jugular bulb, has most commonly been reported [6,7]. Presently, there are no clearly defined guidelines on the medical and/or surgical management of patients presenting with ptCVST [2,8]. Therapy is mainly based on controlling ICP and maintaining normal cerebral perfusion pressure (CPP) [2,8]. The current literature estimates mortality at around 4–8% [3,9]. The mismatch between clinical and imaging findings in patients with TBI and certain risk factors need to raise suspicion of ptCVST. Early recognition of this rare and potentially life-threatening complication is crucial for the effective management of severe TBI patients. Therefore, the purpose of the present case presentation and narrative literature review is to address this important issue for TBI patients and to narratively integrate the various perspectives regarding ptCVST, along with currently available treatment approaches.

2. Case Presentation

This study's case presentation concerns a 66-year-old male patient with an unremarkable past medical history who suffered a moderate traumatic brain injury (TBI) following a 4 m fall. He was immediately transferred to the nearest regional emergency department with an initial Glasgow Coma Scale of 10 out of 15 and mild hemodynamic instability. The patient was intubated, and after primary stabilization, he underwent a full-body computed tomography (CT) scan. Brain and cervical spine CT scans showed several cerebral contusions, pneumocephalus, subdural hematomas, subarachnoid hemorrhage, a fracture of the petrous portion of the temporal bone (Figure 1a,b), and an undisplaced fracture of the second cervical vertebra (Category III of Marshall tomographic score; Injury severity score score of 16). The patient was then transferred to a tertiary hospital intensive care unit with neurosurgical support due to the severity of his condition. Initial ICP measurements (Natus Camino intracranial pressure monitoring catheter, Middleton, WI, USA) were less than 6 mmHg. However, he soon developed several episodes of intracranial hypertension, with ICP measurements as high as 30–35 mmHg, and an external ventricular drain had to be inserted to resolve the condition.

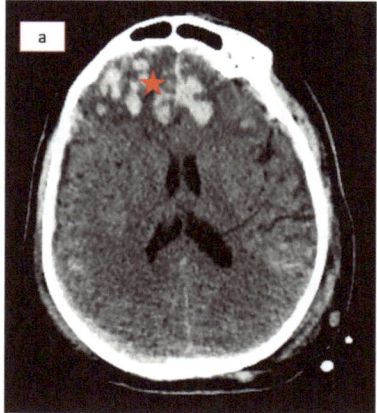 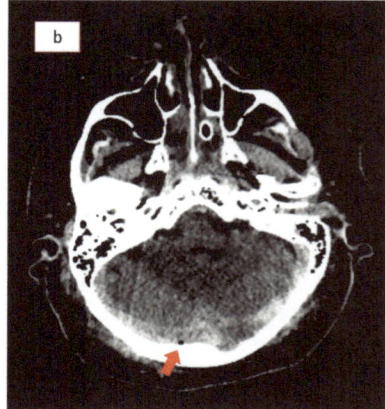

Figure 1. Computed Tomography (CT) scanning upon admission of the patient. (**a**) Hyperdense lesions representing subarachnoid hemorrhage and bilateral cerebral contusions (asterisk). (**b**) Small intracranial collection of air below the occipital bone (arrow).

During his stay in the ICU, the patient also developed a cerebrospinal fluid (CSF) infection, which was successfully treated with broad-spectrum antibiotics. Despite his worsening clinical condition, the following series of brain CT scans showed continuous improvement of the initial traumatic hemorrhagic findings. The mismatch between his clinical and imaging findings raised suspicion for post-traumatic cerebral venous thrombosis, so the patient underwent a CT venography (CTV) on the 14th day of hospitalization. The CTV revealed left transverse sinus and sigmoid sinus thrombosis (Figure 2a,b), which were treated with anticoagulation therapy (high-dose enoxaparin) according to appropriate protocols (Supplementary Figure S1). The patient underwent a tracheostomy due to prolonged mechanical ventilation, and he was then transferred to the Neurosurgical Department, where a gradual neurological improvement was recorded (GCS of 14/15). He was discharged after thirty-eight days of hospitalization with only minor neurological deficits. The patient presented again with cerebrospinal fluid (CSF) rhinorrhea 36 days after discharge, while new CT scans indicated a bone lesion in the roof of the right ethmoid sinus, necessitating lumbar drain catheter insertion with a continuous flow target of 7–10 mL CSF per hour. He was finally discharged after nine days, and no other complications occurred during his following regular follow-ups.

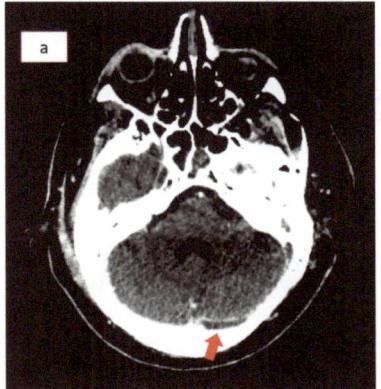 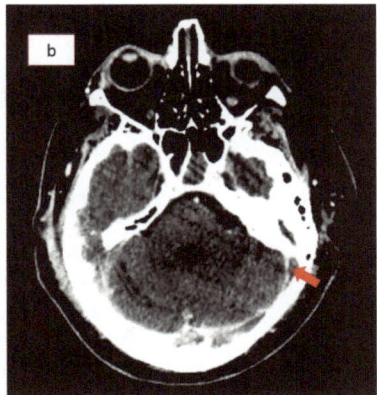

Figure 2. Computed tomography venography (CTV) on the 14th day in the Intensive Care Unit (ICU) revealing thromboses in the (**a**) left transverse and (**b**) sigmoid sinus (red arrows).

3. Discussion

3.1. Epidemiology

CVST, whether post-traumatic or not, constitutes a rare condition, representing 0.5–1% of all strokes, with an incidence of around 2–5 cases per million [10–12]. It is more frequent in younger female patients [9]. Common risk factors include thrombophilia, hormonal-related factors (oral contraceptives, pregnancy), systemic autoimmune diseases or head and neck infections, non-cerebral malignancies, or hematological disorders [10,11]. Traumatic brain injury (TBI) is an underdiagnosed cause of CVST (ptCVST) [1,7,11–15]. The prevalence of ptCVST, even in patients with mild TBI and with suspicion of sinus injury, seems to be around 32%, which is primarily related to a fracture adjacent to the sinus involved [6]. Moreover, the superior sagittal sinus is frequently affected, while multiple sinuses seem to be involved in more than 50% of patients presenting with ptCSVT [16]. Recent reports suggest that ptCVST is more common in adults than pediatric populations, although other studies report similar frequencies of this complication for children and adults [7,14,15].

3.2. Prognosis

According to a multicenter study involving 624 patients, CVST has a 30-day morbidity rate of around 7.7%, regardless of the cause [4]. Furthermore, the 6-month prognosis is generally poor, with one in five patients experiencing unfavorable outcomes [1]. With regard to CVST, mortality rates stand at approximately 5%, mainly attributable to complications related to comorbidities or CVST-related intracranial hemorrhagic events [12]. On the other hand, ptCVST has been linked to lower mean values of initial Glasgow Coma Scale

(GCS) scores, as well as higher scores in the Injury Severity Scoring (ISS) and the Rotterdam CT scoring scales upon admission [4], and has been associated with a mortality rate of less than 10% [4,6]. The prognosis for ptCVST is influenced by various factors, including the patient's age, the specific sinuses affected by CVST, and the ability of the thrombosed or non-thrombosed sinuses to adapt [2,4,16]. Therefore, it seems that the severity of a ptCVST depends on its localization and the influenced anatomical structures [4], while the discrepancy between the clinical course and brain imaging findings of patients might alert clinicians to rule out ptCVST. Notably, pediatric populations may fare better due to increased plasticity of the sinuses in younger ages [2,16].

3.3. Signs and Symptoms

Signs and symptoms of ptCVST are highly heterogeneous and can pose a diagnostic challenge [2,11,16]. Patients who are initially asymptomatic might then develop altered mental status, various types of headaches, visual disturbances, seizures, and cranial nerve deficits, indicating ptCVST [11,12]. A change in the type and intensity of headaches could indicate disease progression or complications, such as subarachnoid or intracranial hemorrhage, venous infarction, cerebral edema, or brain herniation [11]. Therefore, close monitoring for level of consciousness alterations or headaches in the post-TBI course is imperative [11,16]. Moreover, intracranial hypertension is the most common clinical symptom of acute CVST, traumatic or not [17].

3.4. Diagnosis and Radiological Findings

Non-contrast CT (NCCT) is usually the initial diagnostic tool for TBI, but its sensitivity for CVST is only 20–43% [10,18]. Therefore, a normal initial CT scan cannot reliably rule out an active ptCVST [7]. However, certain imaging findings on NCCT, such as skull fractures near a dural sinus, hematoma, intraparenchymal bleeding or hemorrhage of multiple foci, contusions, cerebral edema, pneumocephalus, or signs of venous sinus hyperdensity, such as a cord sign or delta sign, might be suggestive of ptCVST [7,10,11,16]. Thus, early warning clinical symptomatology that is unresponsive to conservative treatment, combined with these imaging findings, should always raise strong suspicion for ptCVST [7,10,11,14] and prompt an emergent contrast-enhanced CTV, which directly detects the venous clot as a filling defect, or a magnetic resonance imaging (MRI)/magnetic resonance venography (MRV) to realize a better description of parenchymal defects as well [19]. Future studies will likely lead to the ultimate guide to patient selection, the best timing, and the appropriate imaging modality for ptCVST diagnosis [7].

Initial imaging studies on asymptomatic patients always carry the risk of not promptly diagnosing a silent ptCVST [20]. However, recent reports indicate that the probability of diagnosing ptCVST increases over time, even 30 days after trauma [7]. Antithrombotic treatments could not be used at the early stages of TBI. Therefore, a proactive, preventive strategy involves performing a standard CT-venography (CTV) within 3–7 days after trauma, when specific indications exist [7]. Delayed imaging studies provide the added benefit of reassessing any new, previously undetected hemorrhagic lesions or signs of ptCVST [7,16]. Following these strategies, a patient with mild TBI and negative imaging after 3–7 days seems to be safe to discharge with regular follow-up visits [7].

3.5. The Anatomy of the Cerebral Venous System

Cerebral veins lack muscular tissue and valves, thus permitting blood to flow bi-directionally [19,21]. The cerebral venous sinus system is responsible for draining deoxygenated blood from the cranial cavity to the cardiovascular circulation [22]. This system consists of superficial and deep cerebral veins [21,23]. The superficial venous system drains into the superior sagittal sinus and the cortical veins, collecting blood from the cortex and outer white matter, whereas the deep venous system comprises the transverse sinuses, the sigmoid sinuses, the straight sinus, deep cerebral veins, and the subependymal and medullary veins draining deeper layers of the white matter and basal ganglia [21,23]. Both systems mostly drain into internal jugular veins [21,23]. The development of collateral circulation creates multiple anastomoses that connect cortical veins and could potentially explain the favorable prognosis of many cases of CVST [19]. The absence of a smooth muscle layer in cerebral veins allows them to generally remain dilated, making patients susceptible to venous air embolism during neurosurgical interventions [24].

3.6. Pathophysiology

The most effective way to understand the clinical entity of CVST is through pathophysiological theories based on Virchow's triad [7]. First, the endothelium's architecture disruption leads to thrombogenic subendothelial tissue exposure, inducing a hypercoagulable state [4,12,19]. The hypercoagulation resulting from blunt head trauma has steadily been identified as an important intravascular predisposing factor for ptCVST [4,12,19]. This has been attributed to the hypercoagulable condition caused by the acceleration of thrombin generation and dysfunction of antithrombin or other anticoagulant mechanisms seen in most trauma patients [2,8]. Moreover, ptCVST can be attributed to stasis caused by factors outside the blood vessels, such as the outer pressure caused by a hematoma, seriously impairing cerebral blood flow [16,19]. Compressive skull fractures, epidural hematomas, and neck collars all induce cerebral blood flow restriction [4,19].

Furthermore, ptCVST leads to venous outflow restriction, resulting in hydrostatic pressure increments of ascending veins and capillaries, ultimately leading to cerebral edema, reduced arterial blood flow, venous infarcts, or blood vessel disruptions and intraparenchymal hemorrhage [16,19]. Venus blood stasis can also induce reduced CSF reabsorption from arachnoid corpuscles that protrude into venous sinuses, deteriorating intracranial hypertension [4,17]. Increased venous pressure finally disrupts the blood–brain barrier (BBB), leading to angiogenic edema, while reduced cerebral blood flow accounts for cytotoxic edema [16,19]. The cytotoxic and angiogenic edema might lead to subsequent infarctions or extension of an existing thrombus [16,19]. Recent research suggests that higher magnitude forces of injury result in more severe thromboses and serious brain damage [7].

3.7. Risk Factors and Etiology

Venous thromboembolism has been associated with female sex, pregnancy, and the use of oral contraceptives [16,25–27]. Other confirmed risk factors are thrombophilia, concomitant neoplasms, infections, postpartum period, systemic diseases, dehydration, intracranial tumors, hypercoagulation, certain medications, trauma, COVID-19 infection, or adenovirus vaccines [1,2,15,16]. However, the cause remains unknown in nearly a third of all cases [15]. Notably, about 20% of CVST cases are associated with thyroid dysfunction [15,28]. The presence of skull fractures or post-traumatic hematomas close to a sinus or the jugular bulb is the predominant risk factor for ptCVST [2,4,15,16]. All types of hematomas are linked to ptCVST, with a recent study demonstrating that nearly all ptCVST cases had subdural, epidural, or both subdural and epidural subarachnoid hemorrhages or contusions [4,16]. Trauma severity also constitutes a serious risk factor for the development of ptCVST, as previously discussed [29].

3.8. Relative Frequency of Venous Sinuses Involved

The frequency of sinuses involved in ptCVST varies in different studies, with recent research demonstrating that ptCVST most commonly involves the superior sagittal sinus and often affects more than one sinus [4,7]. According to a recent study, ptCVST more often affected the anterior, middle, or posterior sections of the superior sagittal sinus, with the entire sinus involved in a portion of cases [16]. The transverse and sigmoid sinuses, or the jugular bulb, also seem to be commonly involved in ptCVST, especially following fractures of the petrous part of the temporal bone, while other usual locations of ptCVST include the internal jugular vein or the deep veins of the brain [2,4,16].

3.9. Non-Surgical Treatment Options

Symptomatic ptCVST, even if accompanied by a secondary hematoma, should be treated according to the American Heart Association, American Stroke Association and European Federation of Neurological Societies guidelines [4,7]. The goal of treatment, besides symptomatic patient relief, should also be prophylaxis against thrombus propagation and complete vessel obstruction, sinus re-tunneling acceleration, the prevention of a new thrombus or embolus formation into the circulation, and intracranial hypertension control [4,7,11]. According to the European Stroke Organization guidelines (2017), low-molecular-weight heparin (LMWH) remains the mainstay of treatment for acute ptCVST [15]. Anticoagulation therapy guidelines for asymptomatic ptCVST have not yet been standardized [1,2,4,7,16].

In cases of ptCVST, it is essential to adopt a distinct clinical approach due to the risk of hematoma rebleeding despite the use of prophylactic anticoagulation doses [14,19,30]. The impact of specific anticoagulation strategies on post-traumatic patients remains quite uncertain, and currently, there are no established guidelines for the treatment of ptCVST [31]. It is necessary to assess whether these strategies offer potential benefits by reducing the risk of further thromboembolic events or if they pose a risk of increased rebleeding [7,19]. Evidence indicates that healthcare providers exhibit hesitancy in initiating anticoagulation therapy for post-traumatic patients [12]. According to a previous study, neurosurgical patients receiving prophylactic doses of LMWH for thromboembolic prophylaxis may face a non-negligible risk of bleeding complications [14]. Certain reports stated that around 43% of patients with ptCVST exhibited substantial clinical improvement and vascular recanalization without anticoagulation therapy [14,30]. Another study reported that hypercoagulation has a minor effect on TBI patient outcomes, suggesting that LMWH should only be considered in selected cases [1]. However, the results of recent meta-analyses advocate the safety of early anticoagulation therapy for traumatic or non-traumatic CVST, regardless of the patient's age [9,14,15,30]. The initiation of enoxaparin following TBI does not seem to worsen clinical outcomes [31,32] and is currently considered a safe intervention in cases where there is no suspected expanding hemorrhage [33]. The use of dose-adjusted intravenous heparin for critical TBI patients has been recommended since the anticoagulant effects of heparin rapidly reverse within a few hours of infusion discontinuation [30]. A recent study revealed minimal adverse events associated with therapeutic anticoagulation in pediatric patients with ptCVST [34]. Epidural hemorrhage or infections can mimic ptCVST by compressing and displacing a sinus, and therefore, using multiple contrast-enhanced imaging planes can aid diagnosis and help avoid complications from anticoagulation [35,36]. Finally, a recent study reported that even prophylactic doses of anticoagulation might lead to hemorrhagic complications and suggested preventive measures with a control CT scan being performed within the first 48 h after the initiation of treatment [6].

3.10. Surgical and Endovascular Treatment

The optimal antithrombotic therapy for ptCVST is a topic of ongoing debate due to the lack of clearly defined guidelines to date [2,16,19]. The primary focus of conservative therapy involves implementing strategies to manage elevated pressure within the skull and restore blood flow to the brain [13,19,24]. Recent reports suggest that mechanical thrombolysis with endovascular interventions could be a promising new treatment option for ptCVST [14,19]. This is especially relevant for patients exhibiting persistent neurological deficits or coma despite receiving antithrombotic therapies and experiencing significant intracranial hemorrhages [1,2,15,16]. Recent studies have emphasized the increasing evidence supporting the safety and effectiveness of combining venous angiogram with intravascular thrombolysis using thrombolytic agents like tissue plasminogen activator (tPA) [14,19]. However, due to the lack of relevant studies, their integration into treatment protocols has yet to be established [2,19]. In cases where patients exhibit persistent signs of intracranial hypertension, surgical decompression may be considered as a rescue therapy [16,19].

Nonetheless, recent research has demonstrated that conservative treatment approaches have produced superior outcomes compared to surgical interventions [11,19].

4. Conclusions

Post-traumatic cerebral venous sinus thrombosis is an uncommon yet potentially life-threatening complication of traumatic brain injury. The presentation of this clinical entity closely resembles that of a severe traumatic brain injury, making it challenging to differentiate. As a result, it is frequently unrecognized. The present research emphasizes the significance of comprehensive planning for contrast-enhanced CT or MRI scans, particularly for TBI patients exhibiting warning clinical signs and concurrent skull fractures near sinuses. Moreover, it is highlighted that the mismatch between clinical and imaging findings in patients with TBI and certain risk factors should raise suspicion for ptCVST. In addition, medical practitioners must carefully weigh the potential complications and contraindications associated with anticoagulant therapy against the risk of untreated patients experiencing thrombus propagation or fatal cerebral edema.

The current state of knowledge necessitates additional investigations to effectively integrate treatment recommendations for this contentious subject into standard clinical procedures. Future algorithms for refractory intracranial hypertension might even suggest that ptCVST be addressed early in the course of TBI and effectively treated with anticoagulation therapy so that a possible subsequent patient deterioration or even a salvage decompressive craniectomy can be prevented. This mainly concerns cases with certain radiological signs, such as fractures or hematomas adjacent to a sinus, or stable radiological signs on sequential imaging studies, which do not fully explain a patient's clinical status.

Supplementary Materials: The following supporting information can be downloaded at: https://www.mdpi.com/article/10.3390/healthcare12171743/s1, Figure S1. Timeline of the patient clinical course during his stay in ICU. TBI: traumatic brain injury; CT: computed tomography; ICP: intracranial pressure; ABX: antibiotic therapy; EVD: external ventricular device; CLABSI: catheter-related blood-stream infection; VAP: ventilator-associated pneumonia; CNS: cerebral nervous system; ptCVST: post-traumatic cerebral venous sinus thrombosis.

Author Contributions: Conceptualization, C.T., A.P., K.N. and E.K.; methodology, C.T., A.T., N.M., S.L. and E.P.; investigation, C.T., G.K., I.K., G.A. and G.V.; resources, N.M., G.K., I.K., G.A. and G.V.; writing—original draft preparation, A.T., M.M., K.N., G.K., I.K., G.A. and G.V.; writing—review and editing, A.T., M.M., K.N., N.M., S.L. and C.T.; visualization, A.T., M.M. and C.T.; supervision, C.T. and E.K.; project administration, C.T. and E.K. All authors have read and agreed to the published version of the manuscript.

Funding: This research received no external funding.

Institutional Review Board Statement: The present report was approved by the Institutional Review Board of the University Hospital of Heraklion, Crete, Greece (Approval Code: 28941/2 October 2023).

Informed Consent Statement: Written informed consent has been obtained from the patient's family to publish this paper.

Data Availability Statement: The data presented in the study are all contained within this article.

Acknowledgments: This manuscript is dedicated to the loving memory of Giannoula Topoliati, who always had a genuine desire to help and eagerly contributed to resolving technical issues for the present report. Moreover, the authors would like to thank this patient's family, who eagerly gave permission for publication. It must also be reported that the present case report was presented at the 19th Panhellenic Conference on Intensive Care in 2023, Athens, Greece.

Conflicts of Interest: The authors declare no conflicts of interest.

References

1. Isan, P.; Mondot, L.; Casolla, B.; Fontaine, D.; Almairac, F. Post-traumatic cerebral venous sinus thrombosis associated with epidural hematoma: A challenging clinical situation. *Neurochirurgie* 2022, 68, e40–e43. [CrossRef] [PubMed]
2. Grangeon, L.; Gilard, V.; Ozkul-Wermester, O.; Lefaucheur, R.; Curey, S.; Gerardin, E.; Derrey, S.; Maltete, D.; Magne, N.; Triquenot, A. Management and outcome of cerebral venous thrombosis after head trauma: A case series. *Rev. Neurol.* 2017, 173, 411–417. [CrossRef]
3. Netteland, D.F.; Sandset, E.C.; Mejlænder-Evjensvold, M.; Aarhus, M.; Jeppesen, E.; Aguiar de Sousa, D.; Helseth, E.; Brommeland, T. Cerebral venous sinus thrombosis in traumatic brain injury: A systematic review of its complications, effect on mortality, diagnostic and therapeutic management, and follow-up. *Front. Neurol.* 2022, 13, 1079579. [CrossRef] [PubMed]
4. Netteland, D.F.; Mejlænder-Evjensvold, M.; Skaga, N.O.; Sandset, E.C.; Aarhus, M.; Helseth, E. Cerebral venous thrombosis in traumatic brain injury: A cause of secondary insults and added mortality. *J. Neurosurg.* 2020, 134, 1912–1920. [CrossRef]
5. Khambholja, J.; Panchal, S.S.; Gami, J.I. A Study of Cerebral Venous Sinus Thrombosis with Special Reference to Newer Risk Predictors. *J. Assoc. Physicians* 2024, 72, 45–56.
6. Meira Goncalves, J.; Carvalho, V.; Cerejo, A.; Polónia, P.; Monteiro, E. Cerebral Venous Thrombosis in Patients with Traumatic Brain Injury: Epidemiology and Outcome. *Cureus* 2024, 16, e55775. [CrossRef] [PubMed]
7. Bokhari, R.; You, E.; Bakhaidar, M.; Bajunaid, K.; Lasry, O.; Zeiler, F.A.; Marcoux, J.; Baeesa, S. Dural Venous Sinus Thrombosis in Patients Presenting with Blunt Traumatic Brain Injuries and Skull Fractures: A Systematic Review and Meta-Analysis. *World Neurosurg.* 2020, 142, 495–505.e3. [CrossRef]
8. Poblete, R.A.; Zhong, C.; Patel, A.; Kuo, G.; Sun, P.Y.; Xiao, J.; Fan, Z.; Sanossian, N.; Towfighi, A.; Lyden, P.D. Post-Traumatic Cerebral Infarction: A Narrative Review of Pathophysiology, Diagnosis, and Treatment. *Neurol. Int.* 2024, 16, 95–112. [CrossRef]
9. Coutinho, J.M.; Zuurbier, S.M.; Stam, J. Declining mortality in cerebral venous thrombosis: A systematic review. *Stroke* 2014, 45, 1338–1341. [CrossRef]
10. Avsenik, J.; Oblak, J.P.; Popovic, K.S. Non-contrast computed tomography in the diagnosis of cerebral venous sinus thrombosis. *Radiol. Oncol.* 2016, 50, 263–268. [CrossRef]
11. Alghamdi, S.R.; Cho, A.; Lam, J.; Al-Saadi, T. Cerebral Venous Sinus Thrombosis in Closed Head Injury: Systematic Review and Meta-analysis. *J. Clin. Neurosci.* 2022, 98, 254–260. [CrossRef] [PubMed]
12. Theologou, R.; Nteveros, A.; Artemiadis, A.; Faropoulos, K. Rare Causes of Cerebral Venus Sinus Thrombosis: A Systematic Review. *Life* 2023, 13, 1178. [CrossRef] [PubMed]
13. Chtara, K.; Bradai, S.; Baccouche, N.; Toumi, N.; Ben Amar, W.; Chelly, H.; Bahloul, M.; Bouaziz, M. Post-traumatic cerebral venous sinus thrombosis in an intensive care unit: A case series of ten patients. *J. Med. Vasc.* 2023, 48, 62–68. [CrossRef]
14. Dobbs, T.D.; Barber, Z.E.; Squier, W.L.; Green, A.L. Cerebral venous sinus thrombosis complicating traumatic head injury. *J Clin. Neurosci.* 2012, 19, 1058–1059. [CrossRef] [PubMed]
15. Gong, S.; Hong, W.; Wu, J.; Xu, J.; Zhao, J.; Zhang, X.; Liu, Y.; Yu, R.-G. Cerebral venous sinus thrombosis caused by traumatic brain injury complicating thyroid storm: A case report and discussion. *BMC Neurol.* 2022, 22, 248. [CrossRef] [PubMed]
16. Harris, L.; Townsend, D.; Ingleton, R.; Kershberg, A.; Uff, C.; O'halloran, P.J.; Offiah, C.; McKenna, G.S. Venous sinus thrombosis in traumatic brain injury: A major trauma centre experience. *Acta Neurochir.* 2021, 163, 2615–2622. [CrossRef]
17. Wei, H.; Jiang, H.; Zhou, Y.; Liu, L.; Zhou, C.; Ji, X. Intracranial hypertension after cerebral venous thrombosis-Risk factors and outcomes. *CNS Neurosci. Ther.* 2023, 29, 2540–2547. [CrossRef]
18. Buyck, P.-J.; Zuurbier, S.M.; Garcia-Esperon, C.; Barboza, M.A.; Costa, P.; Escudero, I.; Renard, D.; Lemmens, R.; Hinteregger, N.; Fazekas, F.; et al. Diagnostic accuracy of noncontrast CT imaging markers in cerebral venous thrombosis. *Neurology* 2019, 92, e841–e851. [CrossRef]
19. Jianu, D.C.; Jianu, S.N.; Dan, T.F.; Munteanu, G.; Copil, A.; Birdac, C.D.; Motoc, A.G.M.; Axelerad, A.D.; Petrica, L.; Arnautu, S.F.; et al. An Integrated Approach on the Diagnosis of Cerebral Veins and Dural Sinuses Thrombosis (a Narrative Review). *Life* 2022, 12, 717. [CrossRef]
20. Jacków-Nowicka, J.; Jagiełło, J.; Dziadkowiak, E.; Bladowska, J.; Sąsiadek, M.; Zimny, A. Acute cerebral venous thrombosis—Still an underdiagnosed pathology in emergency computed tomography of the brain. *Pol. J. Radiol.* 2021, 86, e574–e582. [CrossRef]
21. Kiliç, T.; Akakin, A. Anatomy of cerebral veins and sinuses. *Front. Neurol. Neurosci.* 2008, 23, 4–15. [CrossRef]
22. Bayot, M.L.; Reddy, V.; Zabel, M.K. *Neuroanatomy, Dural Venous Sinuses*; StatPearls Publishing: Treasure Island, FL, USA, 2024.
23. Zuurbier, S.M.; Coutinho, J.M. Cerebral Venous Thrombosis. *Adv. Exp. Med. Biol.* 2017, 906, 183–193. [CrossRef]
24. Prabhakar, H. (Ed.) *Essentials of Neuroanesthesia*; Academic Press: Cambridge, MA, USA, 2017.
25. Pishbin, E.; Ziyaei, M.; Vafadar Moradi, E.; Foroughipour, M.; Javadzadeh, R.; Foroughian, M. Ten-year Causes of Cerebral Venous Sinus Thrombosis in Patients Referred to Ghaem Hospital from 2009 to 2019. *Bull. Emerg. Trauma* 2024, 12, 8–14. [CrossRef]
26. Stančiaková, L.; Brisudová, K.; Škorňová, I.; Bolek, T.; Samoš, M.; Biringer, K.; Staško, J.; Sokol, J. Evaluating Thromboprophylaxis Strategies for High-Risk Pregnancy: A Current Perspective. *Pharmaceuticals* 2024, 17, 773. [CrossRef] [PubMed]
27. de Barros, V.I.P.V.L.; de Oliveira, A.L.M.L.; Nascimento, D.J.D.; Zlotnik, E.; Teruchkin, M.M.; Marques, M.A.; Margarido, P.F.R. Use of hormones and risk of venous thromboembolism. *Rev. Bras. Ginecol. Obstet.* 2024, 46, e-FPS02. [CrossRef]
28. Wakabayashi, T.; Takada, S.; Tsujimoto, Y.; Sadamasa, N.; Taki, W. Cerebral Venous Sinus Thrombosis Associated with Subclinical Hypothyroidism: A Case Report and Literature Review. *Cureus* 2024, 16, e62333. [CrossRef]

29. McGuckin, E.; Ho, K.M.; Honeybul, S.; Stuckey, E.; Song, S. A Prospective Cohort Study Characterizing Incidence of Dural Venous Sinus Thrombosis in Traumatic Brain Injury Patients with Skull Fractures. *World Neurosurg.* **2024**, *184*, e374–e383. [CrossRef] [PubMed]
30. Ochiai, K.; Nishiyama, K. Post-traumatic cerebral sinus thrombosis. *BMJ Case Rep.* **2021**, *14*, e239783. [CrossRef]
31. Samuel, S.; Menchaca, C.; Gusdon, A.M. Timing of anticoagulation for venous thromboembolism after recent traumatic and vascular brain Injury. *J. Thromb. Thrombolysis* **2023**, *55*, 289–296. [CrossRef] [PubMed]
32. Cho, Y.-W.; Scrushy, M.; Zhu, M.; DeAtkine, E.; Wan, B.; Fesmire, A.; Cripps, M.; Park, C. Early administration of high dose enoxaparin after traumatic brain injury. *Eur. J. Trauma Emerg. Surg.* **2023**, *49*, 2295–2303. [CrossRef]
33. Baharvahdat, H.; Ganjeifar, B.; Etemadrezaie, H.; Farajirad, M.; Zabihyan, S.; Mowla, A. Enoxaparin in the treatment of severe traumatic brain injury: A randomized clinical trial. *Surg. Neurol. Int.* **2019**, *10*, 10. [CrossRef] [PubMed]
34. Roth, H.; Ränsch, R.; Kossorotoff, M.; Chahine, A.; Tirel, O.; Brossier, D.; Wroblewski, I.; Orliaguet, G.; Chabrier, S.; Mortamet, G. Post traumatic cerebral sinovenous thrombosis in children: A retrospective and multicenter study. *Eur. J. Paediatr. Neurol.* **2023**, *43*, 12–15. [CrossRef] [PubMed]
35. Irugu, D.-V.-K.; Gupta, M.; Sharma, P.; Ramteke, P.-P.-S.; Sharma, S.-C. Temporal Bone Osteomyelitis in a Child Closely Resembles Lateral Sinus Thrombosis: A Case Report. *Iran. J. Otorhinolaryngol.* **2018**, *30*, 241–245. [PubMed]
36. Singh, S.; Ramakrishnaiah, R.H.; Hegde, S.V.; Glasier, C.M. Compression of the posterior fossa venous sinuses by epidural hemorrhage simulating venous sinus thrombosis: CT and MR findings. *Pediatr. Radiol.* **2016**, *46*, 67–72. [CrossRef]

Disclaimer/Publisher's Note: The statements, opinions and data contained in all publications are solely those of the individual author(s) and contributor(s) and not of MDPI and/or the editor(s). MDPI and/or the editor(s) disclaim responsibility for any injury to people or property resulting from any ideas, methods, instructions or products referred to in the content.

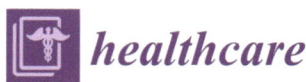

Article

Blood Transfusion Procedure: Assessment of Serbian Intensive Care Nurses' Knowledge

Dragana Simin [1,*], Vladimir Dolinaj [1,2], Branislava Brestovački Svitlica [1,3], Jasmina Grujić [4,5], Dragana Živković [1] and Dragana Milutinović [1]

1. Department of Nursing, Faculty of Medicine, University of Novi Sad, 21000 Novi Sad, Serbia; vladimir.dolinaj@mf.uns.ac.rs (V.D.); branislava.brestovacki@mf.uns.ac.rs (B.B.S.); dragana.zivkovic@mf.uns.ac.rs (D.Ž.); dragana.milutinovic@mf.uns.ac.rs (D.M.)
2. Department of Anesthesia and Intensive Care, University Clinical Centre of Vojvodina, 21000 Novi Sad, Serbia
3. Institute for Child and Youth Health Care of Vojvodina, 21000 Novi Sad, Serbia
4. Department of Transfusiology, Faculty of Medicine, University of Novi Sad, 21000 Novi Sad, Serbia; jasmina.grujic@mf.uns.ac.rs
5. Vojvodina Blood Transfusion Institute, 21000 Novi Sad, Serbia
* Correspondence: dragana.simin@mf.uns.ac.rs

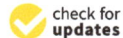

Citation: Simin, D.; Dolinaj, V.; Brestovački Svitlica, B.; Grujić, J.; Živković, D.; Milutinović, D. Blood Transfusion Procedure: Assessment of Serbian Intensive Care Nurses' Knowledge. *Healthcare* **2024**, *12*, 720. https://doi.org/10.3390/healthcare12070720

Academic Editor: Christina Alexopoulou

Received: 26 February 2024
Revised: 18 March 2024
Accepted: 22 March 2024
Published: 25 March 2024

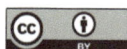

Copyright: © 2024 by the authors. Licensee MDPI, Basel, Switzerland. This article is an open access article distributed under the terms and conditions of the Creative Commons Attribution (CC BY) license (https://creativecommons.org/licenses/by/4.0/).

Abstract: Many patients require administering one or more blood components during hospitalisation in the Intensive Care Unit (ICU). Therefore, nurses' knowledge of who is responsible for immediately administering blood transfusions, monitoring patients, and identifying and managing transfusion reactions is crucial. This cross-sectional descriptive-analytical study aimed to assess the knowledge of ICU nurses in tertiary healthcare institutions about blood transfusion procedures. The questionnaire about the transfusion procedure was designed and reviewed by experts. The questionnaire consisted of 29 items divided into three domains. The scores on the knowledge test ranged from 10 to 27. Generally, 57.7% of nurses had moderate, 23.4% low, and 18.9% high levels of knowledge about the transfusion procedure. Most nurses answered correctly about refreezing fresh frozen plasma, verifying the transfusion product, and identifying the patient. Of the nurses, 91.0% would recognise mild allergic reactions, and 98.2% knew about the supervision of sedated patients. Nurses showed poor knowledge of the length of usage of the same transfusion system for red blood cells, labelling, and transfusion administration in febrile patients. Nurses with higher education and longer working experience had significantly better outcomes ($p = 0.000$) on the knowledge test. Continuous education of ICU nurses on safe transfusion usage is recommended.

Keywords: nurses; transfusion; knowledge; intensive care

1. Introduction

Intensive care units (ICU) are units in which intensive and specialised medical and nursing care to critically ill patients is provided. In these units, an enhanced capacity for monitoring and multiple modalities of physiologic organ support to sustain life through life-threatening organ system insufficiency is enabled [1]. During hospitalisation in the ICU, many patients require the administration of one or more blood components due to ongoing blood loss or haemostatic disorders [2]. When deciding on red blood cell (RBC) transfusion, the following should be taken into account: cause and stage of anaemia, patient comorbidities and age, conditions where there is increased need for oxygen (sepsis), and blood loss [3]. Transfusion trigger is defined as the haemoglobin (Hb) value below which RBC transfusion is indicated. A restrictive transfusion strategy seeks to maintain a lower haemoglobin level (70–90 g/L) with a transfusion trigger when the haemoglobin drops below 70 g/L, whereas a liberal transfusion strategy aims to maintain higher haemoglobin (100–120 g/L), with a threshold for transfusion when haemoglobin drops below 100 g/L [4]. Fresh frozen plasma (FFP) is indicated to substitute coagulation factors in individuals receiving massive transfusions, to reverse warfarin's effect urgently, to treat known coagulation factor deficiency, and in cases of thrombotic thrombocyte thrombocytopenia purpura [5]. Platelet transfusion is usually required in a bleeding patient below a platelet count of $50 \times 10^9/L$ but rarely above $100 \times 10^9/L$. If the values fall between these two, transfusion is considered in cases of platelet dysfunction, ongoing bleeding, and surgeries such as those in the eye and brain [5].

According to the literature, approximately 15–53% of ICU patients receive transfusions [6]. In the United States, in 2021, more than 1.7 million red blood cell units were transfused in ICUs [7]. However, data on the number of administered blood units and the incidence of transfusion in ICU patients in Serbia have not been published.

Blood and blood components perform therapeutic responses and, at the same time, are capable of causing significant adverse effects, which can lead to the deterioration of the critically ill patient's health. The administration of blood products is commonly associated with transfusion reactions, which occur in up to 1 out of every 100 transfusions [8]. Reports show that the incidence of transfusion reactions of RBCs and FFP is 1.7–4.3 per 100,000 transfusions and 62.6 per 100,000 in platelets [9]. The severity of adverse events varies from mild, which could include generalised discomfort, fever, tachycardia, rash, and hypotension, to severe, which could result in anaphylactic reactions and acute haemolytic reaction (AHTR); these could threaten the patient's life [10]. Therefore, transfusion of blood and blood products in the ICU should be considered as administration of any other medication. Thus, before using the blood and blood components in critically ill patients, their use's benefits and risks must be considered [11].

The administration of blood and blood components in the ICU is a multidisciplinary procedure. The multidisciplinary team consists of an anaesthesiologist–intensivist, transfusiologist, and nurse. In the ICU, nurses are responsible for immediate blood transfusions, monitoring patients, and identifying and managing transfusion reactions [12,13].

There are several levels of education for nurses in Serbia. Four-year secondary medical schools provide the first level of nursing education, and higher degrees (bachelor's, master's and doctoral) are obtained at university [14]. Theoretical and practical aspects of the blood transfusion procedure are studied at all levels of education, but to varying degrees. However, regardless of the level of professional training for independent work in the health system, nurses in Serbia must have a license issued by the Chamber of Nurses. The license duration is limited to seven years, and the extension is conditioned by regular attendance of continuing education courses.

Due to the different levels of education of nurses employed in our institution, assessing nurses' knowledge regarding the transfusion of blood and blood products in critically ill patients is of extraordinary importance in ensuring the safety and effectiveness of the transfusion procedures. So far, we know that no similar studies have been carried out in the Republic of Serbia or the southeast region of Europe. Concerning all the issues mentioned above, the study aimed to assess the knowledge of ICU nurses about blood transfusion procedures. In addition, we wanted to identify predictors that might influence their knowledge.

2. Materials and Methods

2.1. Study Design and Settings

A cross-sectional descriptive-analytical study was conducted at the Intensive Care Unit (ICU) of the Clinic of Anesthesia, Intensive Care and Pain Therapy of the University Clinical Center of Vojvodina, in October and November 2022. The University Clinical Center of Vojvodina is one of the regional tertiary healthcare institutions. It provides healthcare services for the area of Vojvodina (a northern province in Serbia) and has 39 beds for intensive care to patients who are critically ill or injured.

The study adhered to Strengthening the Reporting of Observational Studies in Epidemiology (STROBE) guidelines.

2.2. Sample

A purposive sample consisted of Intensive Care Unit nurses. Using sample size software for cross-sectional studies (www.calculator.net; accessed 1 October 2022), it was determined that a sample of 111 nurses was required for a 95% confidence interval, with a margin of error of 0.05.

The criterion for inclusion in the study was that nurses were privileged to direct patient care, had a minimum of 6 months of work experience in the ICU (Figure 1), and voluntarily signed written consent to participate in the study.

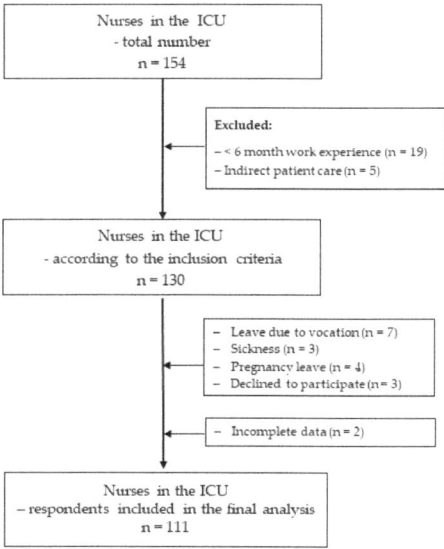

Figure 1. Flowchart summary of data collected from nursing study participants.

2.3. Instrument

The questionnaire on nurses' knowledge of the blood transfusion procedure and a general questionnaire containing data about gender, age, education, and work experience were used as the study instruments.

The researchers designed the questionnaire on nurses' knowledge of the blood transfusion procedure based on the World Health Organization (WHO) Clinical Transfusion Procedure [15], National Guidelines for Clinical Use of Blood [16], and earlier study [17–20]. Before use, the questionnaire was reviewed by a panel of experts consisting of three nurses with academic education, more than ten years of work experience in the ICU, two doctors, one specialist in anaesthesia and intensive care, and one specialist in transfusionology. According to their assessment, the content of the questionnaire was appropriate. The questionnaire consisted of 29 items divided into three domains about nurses' knowledge related to pretransfusion steps (items 1–9) at the beginning of the application of transfusion (items 10–17), and application of transfusion, transfusion reactions (18–29). Nine items (2, 5, 6, 8, 14, 16, 19, 25, and 26) had a true–false answer option, while others were multiple-choice options. Each correct answer is scored with one point. The maximum total score was 29, 9 for the first domain, 8 for the second, and 12 for the third domain of the questionnaire. A score of less than 15 was considered low, 15 to 22 moderate, and a score equal to or greater than 23 indicated a high nurse knowledge level about blood transfusion. The internal consistency was confirmed using the Cronbach's alpha coefficient ($\alpha = 0.72$) and the Spearman–Brown coefficient ($r = 0.79$).

2.4. Data Collection

At the end of the day shift, the researchers distributed paper questionnaires with an information letter and an informed consent form. The nurses who agreed to participate in the study had to sign the informed consent form, and after completing the anonymous questionnaire, nurses had to insert it through the slot into the locked box. In each ICU, nurses are provided an area to fill in the questionnaire independently. They were asked to put down their mobile phones, and the time to complete the questionnaire was not limited.

2.5. Data Analysis

Using IBM statistical software, version 26.0, statistical data processing was performed only for questionnaires where answers were given to all items. Depending on the nature of the variable, descriptive statistics methods were used to determine absolute frequency with appropriate percentages, mean values (M), and standard deviation (SD). The difference between the two groups was compared with the t-test, the Mann–Whitney test, while the one-factor analysis of variance (ANOVA) was used to compare the mean values of several groups. Effect sizes (d and η^2) were calculated to quantify the obtained differences. Standard multiple linear regression analysis was used to predict the factors influencing nurses' knowledge. For all analyses, $p < 0.05$ was considered statistically significant.

2.6. Ethical Consideration

The implementation of this study was approved by the Ethics Committee of the University Clinical Center of Vojvodina (Ref. No. 00-1206/2021). The nurses' consent to participate in the study was obtained following the Declaration of Helsinki

3. Results

3.1. Sociodemographic Characteristics of the Study Sample

Most nurses, 93 (83.8%), were female, and 86 (77.5%) had a secondary medical school diploma. The sociodemographic characteristics of nurses for the whole sample and the level of professional education are shown in Table 1.

Table 1. Sociodemographic characteristics of the study sample (in total and by level of education).

	N (%)		
Variable	All Nurses	SMS	BA
Gender			
Male	18 (16.2)	17 (19.8)	1 (4.0)
Female	93 (83.8)	69 (80.2)	24 (96.0)
Age (years)			
19–28	53 (47.7)	50 (58.1)	3 (12.0)
29–38	36 (32.4)	18 (20.9)	18 (72.0)
39–48	19 (17.1)	15 (17.4)	4 (16.0)
≥49	3 (2.7)	3 (3.5)	0 (0.0)
Work experience			
<1	38 (34.2)	29 (33.7)	9 (36.0)
1–5	36 (32.4)	31 (36.0)	5 (20.0)
≥5	37 (33.3)	26 (30.2)	11 (44.0)

SMS = Secondary medical school; BA = Bachelor's Degree.

3.2. Analysis of Nurses' Knowledge of the Blood Transfusion Procedure

Table 2 shows the distribution of correct answers for each item in the questionnaire.

Table 2. Distribution of nurses' correct answers to items about knowledge related to blood and blood products transfusion procedures.

Items Based on Knowledge of Correct Responses n (%)	
I. Pretransfusion steps	
1. Verification of the medical order for transfusion and patient identification	80 (72.1)
2. Data, time, and place of labelling of blood sample test tubes for pretransfusion tests	26 (23.4)
3. The blood products transportation from the blood bank to the ICU	88 (79.3)
4. The transport of platelet concentrate from the blood bank to the ICU	65 (58.6)
5. Thawing of fresh frozen plasma (FFP)	78 (70.3)
6. Storage of red blood cells (RBCs) in a refrigerator	53 (47.7)
7. The time within unused blood units can be returned to the blood bank	60 (54.1)
8. Refreezing of once-thawed FFP	90 (81.1)
9. Blood product with the highest risk of contamination	41 (36.9)
II. Initiating the transfusion	
10. Verification of the accuracy of the transfusion product and the patient's identity	110 (99.1)
11. Vital signs measured before administration of blood and blood products	79 (71.2)
12. A blood product that does not require a system with an integrated filter	90 (81.1)
13. Peripheral venous cannula (PVC) size for routine transfusion in ICU	80 (72.1)
14. Intravenous solution compatible with blood	99 (89.2)
15. Blood transfusion flow rate at the initiation of administration	59 (53.2)
16. The same transfusion administration set can be applied for the transfusion of 2 to 4 units of RBCs.	50 (45.0)
17. Usage of personal protective equipment—self-protection of the nurses from blood-borne infection	67 (60.4)
III. Administration of transfusion and transfusion reactions	
18. Flow rate of transfusion after the first 15 min from the start of administration	51 (45.9)
19. Monitoring of a sedated patient in the ICU during transfusion	109 (98.2)
20. Time interval of patient observation in the ICU during transfusion administration	64 (57.7)
21. Safe procedure for drug administration during transfusion of blood and blood products	98 (88.3)
22. Mandatory vital signs measured during transfusion of blood and blood products	54 (48.6)
23. The usage of blood transfusion in the ICU in a febrile patient	18 (16.2)
24. Maximum duration of using a transfusion administration set for continuous transfusion	38 (34.2)
25. The maximum time for transfusion of RBCs	48 (43.2)
26. The procedure with the blood and blood products when they were not applied within the stipulated time	82 (73.9)
27. Symptoms and signs of mild allergic transfusion reaction	101 (91.0)
28. Symptoms and signs of an acute haemolytic reaction (AHTR)	51 (45.9)
29. Initial nursing procedures in AHTR	36 (32.4)

Analysis of individual items from the pretransfusion steps domain showed that most correct answers were for the item about refreezing fresh frozen plasma (81.1%). The least correct answers were given to the item about the time and place of filling in the label (23.4%).

Almost all nurses knew how to accurately verify the correctness of the transfusion product and determine the patient's identity at the beginning of the transfusion (99.1%). This item from the domain of initiation of transfusion is also the item with the highest number of correct answers in the entire questionnaire. Also, more than 50% of nurses correctly answered seven out of eight items in this domain. Meanwhile, 45% of nurses were aware that the same transfusion system could be used for 2 to 4 units of red blood cells (RBCs).

The results related to transfusion administration and transfusion reaction show that the least correct answers in this domain, and the entire questionnaire, were to the item about the administration of transfusion in febrile patients in the ICU. In contrast, 91.0% of nurses correctly marked the first signs of a mild allergic reaction, and 98.2% were sure of the supervision required by a sedated patient during a transfusion.

3.3. Total Score on the Knowledge Test

The scores on the knowledge test ranged from 10 to 27 (mean 17.70, SD 4.28). The mean values for each knowledge domain are shown in Table 3.

Table 3. Score on the knowledge test—mean values of the total score and individual domains.

Knowledge TEST Score	Minimum	Maximum	Mean	SD
Total score (0–29)	10.00	27.00	17.70	4.28
Pretransfusion steps (0–9)	2.00	9.00	5.23	1.58
Initiating the transfusion (0–8)	3.00	8.00	5.71	1.32
Administration of transfusion and transfusion reactions (0–12)	3.00	11.00	6.29	1.96

SD = standard deviation.

More than half of the nurses (57.7%) had a moderate level of knowledge, 26 (23.4%) had a low level of knowledge, and 21 nurses had a high level of knowledge about the transfusion procedure. The data in Table 4 indicate that a low level of knowledge was not recorded among nurses with more than five years of work experience and a BA.

Table 4. Distribution of nurses according to levels of knowledge about transfusion and sociodemographic characteristics.

	Knowledge Level		
	Low (0–15)	Moderate (16–22)	High (23–29)
	n (%)	n (%)	n (%)
Total	26 (23.4)	64 (57.7)	21 (18.9)
Gender			
Male	1 (3.8)	17 (26.6)	0 (0.0)
Female	25 (96.2)	47 (73.4)	64 (100)
Educational level			
SMS	26 (100.0)	59 (92.2)	1 (4.8)
BA	0 (0.0)	5 (7.8)	20 (95.2)
Work experience (in years)			
<1	16 (61.5)	16 (25.0)	6 (28.6)
1–5	10 (38.5)	22 (33.4)	4 (19.0)
≥5	0 (0.0)	26 (46.0)	11 (52.4)

SMS = Secondary medical school; BA = Bachelor's Degree.

3.4. Univariate Analysis of Mean Values on the Knowledge Test to the Sociodemographic Characteristics of Nurses

Table 5 shows the differences in mean values on the knowledge test for the entire questionnaire and according to domains. The results of the Mann–Whitney U test showed that the observed differences in all domains of transfusion knowledge to gender were not significant.

On the contrary, the t-test confirmed that the observed higher values of the score on the knowledge test achieved by nurses with higher education differ significantly from those with secondary education. The differences in the scores for the entire questionnaire and in all domains of knowledge related to this sociodemographic characteristic were very significant ($p = 0.00$). Also, Cohen's d values indicate a large effect of education on obtained scores.

Nurses with five or more years of work experience had the best knowledge on the test. The significance of this difference was not confirmed by a one-factor analysis of variance for the pretransfusion steps domain ($p = 0.425$). At the same time, the observed differences for the total score and other knowledge domains were very significant ($p = 0.00$); according to Cohen's d values, they had a large effect.

Table 5. Nurses' knowledge test scores differences to nurses' sociodemographic characteristics.

Sociodemographic Characteristic	Total Score				Pretransfusion Steps				Initiating the Transfusion				Administration of Transfusion and Transfusion Reactions			
	M ±SD	U	p	r	M ±SD	U	p	r	M ±SD	U	p	r	M ±SD	U	p	r
Gender		835.00	0.987	ns		707.00	0.288	ns		654.00	0.132	ns		797.00	0.746	ns
Male	17.72 ± 1.93				4.89 ± 1.13				6.16 ± 1.04				6.22 ± 1.11			
Female	17.69 ± 4.61				5.30 ± 1.65				5.62 ± 1.35				6.31 ± 2.10			
Educational level	M ±SD	t (df)	p	d	M ±SD	t (df)	p	d	M ±SD	t (df)	p	d	M ±SD	t (df)	p	d
		11.022 (109)	0.000	0.53 *		11.053 (109)	0.000	0.53 *		4.504 (109)	0.000	0.16 *		8.086 (109)	0.000	0.38 *
SMS	16.03 ± 3.15				4.62 ± 1.07				5.43 ± 1.32				5.65 ± 1.57			
BA	23.44 ± 2.14				7.36 ± 1.15				6.68 ± 0.75				8.51 ± 1.53			
Work experience (in years)	M ±SD	F (df)	p	η²	M ±SD	F (df)	p	η²	M ±SD	F (df)	p	η²	M ±SD	F (df)	p	η²
		9.201 (110)	0.000	0.15 *		0.863 (110)	0.425	ns		14.467 (110)	0.000	0.21 *		8.636 (110)	0.000	0.14 *
<1	16.63 ± 5.17				5.11 ± 1.99				5.31 ± 1.56				5.82 ± 1.82			
1–5	16.47 ± 3.65				5.08 ± 1.27				5.25 ± 0.94				5.75 ± 1.76			
≥5	20.00 ± 2.71				5.51 ± 1.37				6.56 ± 0.93				7.32 ± 1.93			

M = mean; SD = standard deviation; U = Mann–Whitney test; p-value; r-value; ns = not significant; t = t-test; df = degrees of freedom; d = Cohen's d indicator (* large effect); F = ANOVA; η² = partial eta squared; SMS = Secondary medical school; BA = Bachelor's Degree.

3.5. Standard Multiple Regression Analysis of the Effect of Sociodemographic Characteristics on the Knowledge Test Score

The results obtained by standard multiple regression analysis indicate that our model, which included the level of education and work experience, explains 60.6% of the variance in the total score on the transfusion knowledge test (Table 6). Although both variables make a statistically significant contribution, the highest contribution is made by the level of education (Beta = 0.710).

Table 6. Standard multiple regression model for the prediction of the total score.

	Unstandardised Coefficient		Standardised Coefficient	t-Value	p-Value	Correlations Part	F	p-Value
	ß	SE	Beta					
Constant	5.926	0.986		6.010	0.000			
Level Education	7.237	0.617	0.710	11.731	0.000	0.708	83.152	0.000
Work experience	1.461	0.314	0..282	4.661	0.000	0.281		

ß = coefficient; SE = Standard Error; F = ANOVA.

4. Discussion

Blood transfusion is a common procedure in the ICU. Many factors contribute to ICU patients being frequent recipients of allogeneic blood transfusions [11]. During their ICU stay, 15% to 53% of patients receive a transfusion [6]. The results of a recent international prospective study conducted in 30 countries where data from 233 ICUs were analysed showed that 25% of patients received one or more units of red blood cells (RBCs) [7]. Proper use of blood transfusion and blood derivatives saves lives and improves the health of many people [15]. Like any therapeutic procedure and transfusion, there are several potential risks to patient safety. The basis for minimising these risks is that the transfusion is applied by trained and experienced personnel and by rigorous adherence to the entire procedure process [21].

More than half of the nurses in this study had a moderate level of knowledge about blood transfusion. Earlier studies also showed that nurses' knowledge of this procedure was low or moderate [12,13,17,18,20,22–26]. Since transfusion of blood and blood products is a multistage procedure, our studies and those mentioned above aim to be used to identify risky parts of the transfusion process and at-risk populations of blood recipients to ensure safe blood administration in intensive care units.

One of the first steps in safely and properly administering transfusion involves providing the right blood to the right patient at the right time [15,16]. The results of our study showed that almost a third of nurses have adequate knowledge regarding medical orders and patient identification verification. However, only 26 (23.4%) of our nurses marked all the data that the label must contain and that the data on the label should be filled in at the patient's bedside immediately after taking the blood sample. This step in the transfusion procedure is extremely important because of the risk that the patient's blood sample will end up in the wrong sample test tube. The sample test tube should not be labelled before taking the sample [15]. When the blood in the sample test tube is not the blood of the patient whose information is on the label, it can lead to fatal outcomes due to the transfusion of ABO-incompatible blood [27].

The application of information technology can significantly contribute to reducing this and other errors related to blood transfusion [12]. Currently, the barcoding system is commonly used but is slowly being replaced by a radio-frequency identification tag system. Unfortunately, the price often limits their application [27]. The financial aspects of the institution where the study was conducted significantly prevent the implementation of many modern technologies in the entire clinical care process. The application of barcode technology started a few years ago in certain areas of laboratory diagnostics. However, this system has not yet covered all segments of patient care during hospitalisation. The impact of the human factor can be reduced by applying modern technologies, but they alone cannot completely remove all risks [6,27]. At the same time, a project implemented in the Basque Country showed that regional information systems that generate all relevant information in all stages of the blood transfusion process can significantly increase patient safety and transfusion efficiency [28]. Considering the results obtained with this research of our ICU nurses and our institution's technical (in)ability in order to reduce the risk of fatal errors in pretransfusion time, multiple interventions should be undertaken, such as education of nursing staff, raising awareness about the causes and impact of human error on patient safety, and the rigorous control of the superior nurses [27].

The nurses in our study had a high level of knowledge about transporting blood from the blood bank to the ICU (79.3%). However, slightly more than half of the nurses (58.6%) stated that constant agitation is necessary when transporting concentrated platelets longer than 2 h. Such answers can perhaps be explained by the fact that the service for the blood bank and the ICU is not far away and that the transfer does not take more than 15 min. At the same time, it should not be overlooked that only a third of the nurses marked concerted platelets as the derivative with the highest risk for infection. Namely, to preserve the function of platelets, they are not cooled but stored at a temperature of 22 °C to 24 °C, which increases the risk of proliferation of bacteria and other microorganisms [15,16].

The obtained results suggest that future activities should increase patient safety during blood transfusion and focus on nursing interventions regarding healthcare-acquired infection (HAI). Moreover, this aspect requires special attention because the risk of HAIs is twice as high in ICU patients compared to patients from other clinical departments [29]. The high prevalence of invasive procedures and therapeutic modalities, the use of immunosuppressive drugs, and the presence of comorbidities significantly contribute to the fact that patients in the ICU have this level of risk of HAI [30]. According to Edwardson [29], blood transfusion is one of the factors that can increase the risk of HAIs in the ICU. Nurses can significantly contribute to the implementation of HAI prevention measures in this, as well as in other domains of patient care in the ICU. Namely, of all multidisciplinary team members in the ICU, nurses are more often in direct contact with the patient [30].

Analysis of responses of our ICU nurses about how to thaw FFP and refreeze once-thawed FFP showed that the nurses in this study had a high level of knowledge. However, our nurses, as well as nurses in several other studies, did not have enough knowledge about storing other blood products and returning unused products to the blood bank [18–20,31–33]. Freixo et al. [31], in a critical analysis of the nurses' responses, state that this can negatively affect the quality of blood products and the adequate management of supplies. Namely, two crucial rules for the storage of blood products are the 30 min rule, the period in which the product must be used since it is not stored in a temperature-controlled environment, and the 4 h rule, the time within which the transfusion should be completed [15].

The nurses in our study knew the principles of good practices related to verifying the blood product's correctness and the patient's identity immediately before the start of the transfusion. Namely, almost all nurses (99.1%) correctly marked all necessary elements of verification and identification. The same results were obtained in the studies of Uzun et al. [26]. The literature data indicate that these procedures may be absent in patients with active bleeding and when nurses start the transfusion after the shift [23,24]. Also, the reason for the incorrect answer regarding blood product verification was the practice in which only one nurse performed the check [19]. These findings indicate that potentially skipping certain procedures would increase the risk for the safe application of transfusion; that is, the chance that the right blood will not be given to the right patient is increased [23].

Although most patients in the ICU have a central venous catheter in place, the peripheral venous cannula (PVC) is also a means of providing vascular access through which transfusion to critically ill patients can be administered. Based on several criteria, nurses independently decide on the size of the PVC which will be placed in the patient. The recommendation for the application of routine transfusion of most blood products is that the size of PVC should be from 20 to 24 gauge (G), while for rapid transfusion, the recommendation is that the PVC should be of a larger diameter, size 18 to 20 G [34]. For routine use of RBCs, a PVC size of 20 to 22 G is recommended due to the reduced risk of haemolysis, and for rapid transfusion, RBC size should be from 16 to 18 G [15].

More than two-thirds of our ICU nurses correctly answered the item about the size of the PVC in routine transfusion. The answers of other nurses were consistent with those of nurses in studies where a few nurses gave the correct answer to this item [20,26]. Namely, in our study, as in studies of Jogi et al. and Uzun, further analysis determined that nurses opted for cannulas of a significantly larger diameter, even in a routine, not an emergency, transfusion. However, although a PVC with a larger diameter will enable faster transfusion flow, at the same time, it will significantly increase the risk of mechanical phlebitis [34].

The results of our study indicate that ICU nurses and nurses from other clinical departments generally have a high level of knowledge about solutions compatible with blood products and how to administer drugs during transfusion. This finding is similar to previously published research [17,19,23,24,26].

Most standard administrative transfusion sets have integrated filters from 170 to 260 microns, with a maximum capacity of 4 units of RBCs [34]. Most care systems and transfusion administration sets are replaced following the manufacturer's recommendations. In order to prevent the proliferation of microorganisms, the general recommendation is to change the blood administration set for continuous transfusion every 12 h [15,34]. The nurses' knowledge in our study was deficient about blood administration set replacement when administering 2 to 4 units of RBCs and during continuous transfusion. Namely, most nurses who did not give the correct answer (from 2 to 4 units of RBCs and 12 h in case of continuous transfusion) indicated that regardless of the number of units the patient receives, a new blood administration set is used for each unit of blood product. From a financial perspective, this practice is questionable because it additionally increases the costs of the patient's stay in the ICU. At the same time, it is also questionable from the aspect of the risk of HAI because with each replacement of the set, the number of manipulations with the luer extension of the vascular access device (PVC or central venous catheter) increases.

If signs of transfusion reactions do not appear during the first 15 min of transfusion administration, the flow rate of 50 mL/h is increased to meet the total administration time [15,34]. In our study, nurses had a low level of knowledge on items about blood transfusion flow rate. Similar results were obtained in previously published studies [17,18,20,22]. Also, more than half of the nurses in our study did not correctly answer the item about the maximum time required for RBC administration. In contrast, a significantly larger number of them (73.9%) answered that if the time for blood administration has expired (duration of transfusion longer than 4 h), the administration of blood should be stopped, and the anaesthesiologist–intensivist should decide whether to prescribe another unit.

It is well known that in the early stage of deterioration of the patient's condition, as a response to inadequate oxygenation, the frequency of respiration and pulse increases, while the values of peripheral oxygen saturation (SpO2) and arterial blood pressure are without significant changes [35].

We find that the nurses' level of knowledge regarding assessing vital signs at the beginning of transfusion administration (71.2%) and monitoring unconscious patients (72.1%) was satisfactory. However, they had a significantly lower level of knowledge about the observation time interval (57.7%) and the mandatory vital signs monitored during transfusion (48.6%). Since this was a multiple-choice item, we observed through detailed analysis that respiration rate was often not recognised as a vital function monitored during transfusion. According to the literature data, although it can contribute to the early recognition of dehydration in a patient, nurses often omit the assessment of breathing in clinical practice [36]. Such practice increases the risk that the patient's deterioration is not recognised in time.

The lowest number of correct answers we received in this study were on the item about administering a transfusion to a febrile patient. This rate of correct responses may have been attributed to the fact that nurses do not consider decision-making about therapeutic procedures as their responsibility, nor collaborative, but solely the physician's responsibility.

Adequate patient observation and monitoring of vital signs in all transfusion steps contribute to early detection and effective treatment of transfusion reactions [15]. Most of our nurses knew that urticarial rash usually occurs with a mild allergic reaction. However, regarding acute haemolytic reaction (AHTR), a significantly lower number of nurses answered correctly. Namely, 51 (45.9%) nurses correctly marked the symptoms and signs of AHTR. At the same time, every third nurse (32.4%) answered correctly about the nursing management of this serious and potentially life-threatening complication. The implication of the authors of studies where nurses had a knowledge deficit in the domain of the AHTR is that additional, periodically repetitive education is necessary [17,19]. A similar conclusion was made in the study of Uzun, where the results showed that the nursing management of transfusion reactions was well known to nurses [26]. Such a conclusion is not surprising because patient safety is a key aspect of all procedures during transfusion [15].

According to our results, nurses' education level is a predictor of success on the transfusion knowledge test: nurses with a higher level of education had significantly better knowledge about transfusion compared to nurses with a lower level of education. This correlates with earlier conducted research [13,19,22,25]. Our findings showed that none of the ICU nurses with a higher level of education had a low level of knowledge about transfusion. Such results are not surprising from the perspective of the scope of the content of the programs' curricula at different levels of education.

Encan and Dubey reported that nurses with more work experience had better knowledge about transfusion [19,22]. We obtained similar results. Working experience was a significant predictor of transfusion knowledge in our sample. Nurses with five or more years of work experience had the best knowledge, followed by those with less than one year and at least one to five years of work experience. In contrast, Panchawagh [32] and colleagues determined that nurses with one to five years of work experience had significantly better knowledge. In the same study, nurses with more than five years of experience had the lowest level of knowledge. The authors cite forgetting fundamental knowledge as one of the possible causes [32].

Inadequate knowledge is only one of the barriers to implementing safe transfusion practices. Hijji et al. [18] suggest that for the maximum application of this practice, it is necessary to overcome both personal obstacles by developing positive attitudes and many organisational obstacles, such as the number of nurses and material resources. Smith et al. [37] confirmed that carefully designed structured transfusion education programs have long-term positive effects. However, it was revealed that nurses' knowledge levels did not decrease over time, but their attitudes about safe transfusion practice changed positively.

Limitations

This study has strengths, such as providing significant data on ICU nurses' transfusion knowledge, having a sufficient sample, and having a questionnaire with many items that panel experts revised, but it has certain weaknesses. First, the study was conducted in only one institution with a cross-sectional design, which limits the generalisation of the results. Also, although the study's authors tried to include as many transfusion-related procedures of ICU nurses as possible in the questionnaire, some procedures may not be included.

5. Conclusions

The results of this study indicate that most Serbian ICU nurses had a moderate or low knowledge of transfusion. At the same time, a high deficit of knowledge was determined for the procedures of marking the blood sample tube, the rate of transfusion flow, the time of replacement of the transfusion administration set, and the procedures of observation and nursing management of transfusion reactions. Nurses with a higher level of education and longer working experience had significantly better knowledge. The results can be the basis for creating structured continuous education, which would increase knowledge, improve practice, and reduce risks to patient safety during the transfusion procedure.

Author Contributions: Conceptualisation, D.M. and D.S.; methodology, D.S., V.D. and D.M.; investigation, V.D., J.G., B.B.S. and D.S.; formal analysis, D.S. and D.M.; writing—original draft preparation, D.S. and D.M.; writing—review and editing, V.D., J.G., D.Ž. and B.B.S.; visualisation, D.S.; supervision, J.G. and D.M. All authors have read and agreed to the published version of the manuscript.

Funding: This research received no external funding.

Institutional Review Board Statement: The implementation of this study was approved by the Ethics Committee of the University Clinical Center of Vojvodina (Ref. No. 00-1206/31.12.2019). The nurses' consent to participate in the study was obtained in accordance with the Declaration of Helsinki.

Informed Consent Statement: Informed consent was obtained from all subjects involved in the study.

Data Availability Statement: All data relevant to the study are included in the article.

Acknowledgments: We would like to thank all the nurses who participated in this research.

Conflicts of Interest: The authors declare no conflicts of interest.

References

1. Marshall, J.C.; Bosco, L.; Adhikari, N.K.; Connolly, B.; Diaz, J.V.; Dorman, T.; Fowler, R.A.; Meyfroidt, G.; Nakagawa, S.; Pelosi, P.; et al. What is an intensive care unit? A report of the task force of the World Federation of Societies of Intensive and Critical Care Medicine. *J. Crit. Care* **2017**, *37*, 270–276. [CrossRef]
2. Neuenfeldt, F.S.; Weigand, M.A.; Fischer, D. Coagulopathies in Intensive Care Medicine: Balancing Act between Thrombosis and Bleeding. *J. Clin. Med.* **2021**, *10*, 5369. [CrossRef] [PubMed]
3. Goel, R.; Patel, E.U.; Cushing, M.M.; Frank, S.M.; Ness, P.M.; Takemoto, C.M.; Vasovic, L.V.; Sheth, S.; Nellis, M.E.; Shaz, B.; et al. Association of Perioperative Red Blood Cell Transfusions With Venous Thromboembolism in a North American Registry. *JAMA Surg.* **2018**, *153*, 826–833. [CrossRef]
4. Estcourt, L.J.; Malouf, R.; Trivella, M.; Fergusson, D.A.; Hopewell, S.; Murphy, M.F. Restrictive versus liberal red blood cell transfusion strategies for people with haematological malignancies treated with intensive chemotherapy or radiotherapy, or both, with or without haematopoietic stem cell support. *Cochrane Database Syst. Rev.* **2017**, *1*, CD011305. [CrossRef] [PubMed]
5. Liumbruno, G.; Bennardello, F.; Lattanzio, A.; Piccoli, P.; Rossetti, G.; Italian Society of Transfusion Medicine and Immunohaematology (SIMTI) Work Group. Recommendations for the transfusion of plasma and platelets. *Blood Transfus.* **2009**, *7*, 132–150. [CrossRef] [PubMed]
6. Nayeri, N.D.; Nadali, J.; Divani, A.; Hatefimoadab, N. Ways To Enhance Blood Transfusion Safety: A Systematic Review. *Florence Nightingale J. Nurs.* **2022**, *30*, 288–300. [CrossRef] [PubMed]
7. Raasveld, S.J.; de Bruin, S.; Reuland, M.C.; Oord, C.v.D.; Schenk, J.; Aubron, C.; Bakker, J.; Cecconi, M.; Feldheiser, A.; Meier, J.; et al. Blood Cell Transfusion in the Intensive Care Unit. *JAMA* **2023**, *330*, 1852–1861. [CrossRef] [PubMed]
8. Delaney, M.; Wendel, S.; Bercovitz, R.S.; Cid, J.; Cohn, C.; Dunbar, N.M.; O Apelseth, T.; Popovsky, M.; Stanworth, S.J.; Tinmouth, A.; et al. Transfusion reactions: Prevention, diagnosis, and treatment. *Lancet* **2016**, *388*, 2825–2836. [CrossRef]
9. Sandler, S.G.; Vassallo, R.R. Anaphylactic transfusion reactions. *Transfusion* **2011**, *51*, 2265–2266. [CrossRef]
10. Eder, A.F.; Dy, B.A.; Perez, J.M.; Rambaud, M.; Benjamin, R.J. The residual risk of transfusion-related acute lung injury at the American Red Cross (2008–2011): Limitations of a predominantly male-donor plasma mitigation strategy. *Transfusion* **2013**, *53*, 1442–1449. [CrossRef]
11. Shander, A.; Javidroozi, M.; Lobel, G. Patient Blood Management in the Intensive Care Unit. *Transfus. Med. Rev.* **2017**, *31*, 264–271. [CrossRef] [PubMed]
12. da Silva, K.F.N.; Duarte, R.D.; Floriano, D.R.; Andrade, L.F.; Tavares, J.L.; Félix, M.M.d.S.; Zuffi, F.B.; Pires, P.D.S.; Barbosa, M.H. Blood transfusion in Intensive Care Units: Knowledge of the nursing team. *Av. En. Enfermería* **2017**, *35*, 313–323. [CrossRef]
13. Duarte, R.D.; da Silva, K.F.N.; dos Santos Félix, M.M.; Tavares, J.L.; Zuffi, F.B.; Barbosa, M.H. Knowledge about blood transfusion in a critical unit of a teaching hospital. *Biosci. J.* **2017**, *33*, 788–798. [CrossRef]
14. Milutinović, D.; Lovrić, R.; Simin, D. Interprofessional education and collaborative practice: Psychometric analysis of the Readiness for Interprofessional Learning Scale in undergraduate Serbian healthcare student context. *Nurse Educ. Today* **2018**, *65*, 74–80. [CrossRef] [PubMed]
15. World Health Organization. Educational Modules on Clinical Use of Blood. 2021. Available online: https://iris.who.int/bitstream/handle/10665/350246/9789240033733-eng.pdf (accessed on 12 March 2022).
16. Milosavljević, T. *Postupak Primene Krvnih Komponenti i Transfuzijske Reakcije: Nacionalni Vodič: Republička Stručna Komisija za Transfuziologiju/The Procedure for Administration of Blood Components and Transfusion Reactions: A National Guide*; Expert Commission for Transfusiology of the Republic of Serbia: Beograd, Serbia, 2005; pp. 2–59.
17. Hijji, B.; Parahoo, K.; Hussein, M.M.; Barr, O. Knowledge of blood transfusion among nurses. *J. Clin. Nurs.* **2012**, *22*, 2536–2550. [CrossRef] [PubMed]

18. Hijji, B.M.; Oweis, A.E.; Dabbour, R.S. Measuring knowledge of blood transfusion: A survey of Jordanian nurses. *Am. Int. J. Contemp. Res.* **2012**, *2*, 77–94.
19. Encan, B.; Akin, S. Knowledge of Blood Transfusion Among Nurses. *J. Contin. Educ. Nurs.* **2019**, *50*, 176–182. [CrossRef]
20. Jogi, I.E.; Mohanan, N.; Nedungalaparambil, N.M. Bedside blood transfusion—What nurses know and perform: A cross-sectional study from a tertiary-level cancer hospital in rural Kerala. *Asia Pac. J. Oncol. Nurs.* **2021**, *8*, 197–203. [CrossRef]
21. Brown, M.; Brown, C. Improving nurses' blood transfusion knowledge and skills. *Br. J. Nurs.* **2023**, *32*, 522–525. [CrossRef]
22. Dubey, A.; Sonker, A.; Chaudhary, R. Evaluation of health care workers' knowledge and functioning of blood centres in north India: A questionnaire based survey. *Transfus. Apher. Sci.* **2013**, *4*, 565–570. [CrossRef]
23. Lee, S.L.E.; Rahim, A.N.A.; Azdiana, S.; Din, T.S.A. Knowledge of blood transfusion among nurses at hospital pulau pinang: Nursing responsibilities and patient management related to transfusion reactions. *Educ. Med. J.* **2016**, *8*, 47–56. [CrossRef]
24. Noor, N.H.M.; Saad, N.H.; Khan, M.; Hassan, M.N.; Ramli, M.; Bahar, R.; Yusoff, S.M.; Iberahim, S.; Ab Rahman, W.S.W.; Zulkafli, Z.; et al. Blood Transfusion Knowledge among Nurses in Malaysia: A University Hospital Experience. *Int. J. Environ. Res. Public Health* **2021**, *18*, 11194. [CrossRef]
25. Gaur, R.; Mudgal, S.K.; Suyal, N.; Sharma, S.K.; Agarwal, R.; Raj, R.; Jitender, C. Nurses and nursing students' knowledge regarding blood transfusion: A comparative cross-sectional study. *J. Integr. Nurs.* **2022**, *4*, 137–144. [CrossRef]
26. Uzun, B.; Yılmaz, V.; Göklü, S.; Şahbaz, U.; Güvel, H. Blood transfusion knowledge levels of nurses in İzmir Atatürk training and research Hospital, turkey. *Transfus. Clin. Biol.* **2024**, *S1246-7820*, 00002–00008. [CrossRef]
27. Bolton-Maggs, P.H.B.; Wood, E.M.; Wiersum-Osselton, J.C. Wrong blood in tube—Potential for serious outcomes: Can it be prevented? *Br. J. Haematol.* **2015**, *168*, 3–13. [CrossRef]
28. Vesga, M.A.; Azkárate, M. Information systems for a blood transfusion regional network. *VOXS* **2021**, *16*, 231–238. [CrossRef]
29. Edwardson, S.; Cairns, C. Nosocomial infections in the ICU. *Anaesth. Intensive Care Med.* **2019**, *20*, 14–18. [CrossRef]
30. Blot, S.; Ruppé, E.; Harbarth, S.; Asehnoune, K.; Poulakou, G.; Luyt, C.-E.; Rello, J.; Klompas, M.; Depuydt, P.; Eckmann, C.; et al. Healthcare-associated infections in adult intensive care unit patients: Changes in epidemiology, diagnosis, prevention and contributions of new technologies. *Intensive Crit. Care Nurs.* **2022**, *70*, 103227. [CrossRef]
31. Freixo, A.; Matos, I.; Leite, A.; Silva, A.; Bischoff, F.; Carvalho, M.; Monteiro, C.; Ferreira, A.; Fernandes, S.; Lemos, N.; et al. Nurses knowledge in Transfusion Medicine in a Portuguese university hospital: The impact of an education. *Blood Transfus.* **2017**, *15*, 49–52. [CrossRef]
32. Panchawagh, S.J.; Melinkeri, S.; Panchawagh, M.J. Assessment of Knowledge and Practice of Blood Transfusion Among Nurses in a Tertiary Care Hospital in India. *Indian J. Hematol. Blood Transfus.* **2020**, *36*, 393–398. [CrossRef]
33. Louw, L.D.; Grobbelaar, J.; Henn, L.; van Zyl, L.; Wernich, C.; Wessels, P.-L.; Setlogelo, O.; Joubert, G.; Barrett, C. Management of blood products: Nursing knowledge and practices at an academic hospital. *Transfus. Apher. Sci.* **2021**, *60*, 102971. [CrossRef]
34. Gorski, L.A.M.; Hadaway, L.M.; Hagle, M.E.P.; Broadhurst, D.M.; Clare, S.M.; Kleidon, T.M.; Meyer, B.M.P.; Nickel, B.A.-C.; Rowley, S.M.; Sharpe, E.D.; et al. Infusion therapy standards of practice, 8th Edition. *J. Infus. Nurs.* **2021**, *44*, S1–S224. [CrossRef]
35. Mok, W.Q.; Wang, W.; Liaw, S.Y. Vital signs to detect deterioration. *Int. J. Nurs. Pract.* **2015**, *21* (Suppl. S2), 91–98. [CrossRef]
36. Kelly, C. Respiratory rate 1: Why measurement and recording are crucial. *Nurs. Times* **2018**, *114*, 23–24.
37. Smith, A.; Gray, A.; Atherton, I.; Pirie, E.; Jepson, R. Does time matter? An investigation of knowledge and attitudes following blood transfusion training. *Nurse Educ. Pract.* **2014**, *14*, 176–182. [CrossRef]

Disclaimer/Publisher's Note: The statements, opinions and data contained in all publications are solely those of the individual author(s) and contributor(s) and not of MDPI and/or the editor(s). MDPI and/or the editor(s) disclaim responsibility for any injury to people or property resulting from any ideas, methods, instructions or products referred to in the content.

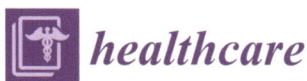

Article

Personality Traits, Burnout, and Psychopathology in Healthcare Professionals in Intensive Care Units—A Moderated Analysis

Varvara Pakou [1], Dimitrios Tsartsalis [2,3,*], Georgios Papathanakos [1], Elena Dragioti [2], Mary Gouva [2] and Vasilios Koulouras [1]

[1] Intensive Care Unit, University Hospital of Ioannina, University of Ioannina, 45500 Ioannina, Greece; varvarapak@uoi.gr (V.P.); gppthan@icloud.com (G.P.); vpkoulouras@yahoo.gr (V.K.)
[2] Laboratory of Psychology of Patients, Families & Health Professionals, Department of Nursing, School of Health Sciences, University of Ioannina, 45500 Ioannina, Greece; dragioti@uoi.gr (E.D.); gouva@uoi.gr (M.G.)
[3] Department of Clinical Physiology, Sundsvall Hospital, 85643 Sundsvall, Sweden
* Correspondence: dtsartsalis@gmail.com; Tel.: +46-7352-97599

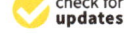

Citation: Pakou, V.; Tsartsalis, D.; Papathanakos, G.; Dragioti, E.; Gouva, M.; Koulouras, V. Personality Traits, Burnout, and Psychopathology in Healthcare Professionals in Intensive Care Units—A Moderated Analysis. *Healthcare* 2024, *12*, 587. https://doi.org/10.3390/healthcare12050587

Academic Editor: Christina Alexopoulou

Received: 27 January 2024
Revised: 24 February 2024
Accepted: 1 March 2024
Published: 4 March 2024

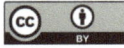

Copyright: © 2024 by the authors. Licensee MDPI, Basel, Switzerland. This article is an open access article distributed under the terms and conditions of the Creative Commons Attribution (CC BY) license (https://creativecommons.org/licenses/by/4.0/).

Abstract: This study explored the associations between personality dimensions, burnout, and psychopathology in healthcare professionals in intensive care units (ICUs). This study further aimed to discern the differences in these relationships when considering the variables of critical care experience (less than 5 years, 5–10 years, and more than 10 years), profession (nurses versus intensivists), and the urban size of the city where the ICU is located (metropolitan cities versus smaller urban cities). This cross-sectional investigation's outcomes are based on data from 503 ICU personnel, including 155 intensivists and 348 nurses, in 31 ICU departments in Greece. Participants underwent a comprehensive assessment involving a sociodemographic questionnaire, the Eysenck Personality Questionnaire (EPQ), the Maslach Burnout Inventory (MBI), and the Symptom Checklist-90 (SCL-90). To analyze the interplay among critical care experience, burnout status, and psychopathology, a moderation analysis was conducted with personality dimensions (i.e., psychoticism, extraversion, and neuroticism) serving as the mediator variable. Profession and the urban size of the ICU location were considered as moderators influencing these relationships. Male healthcare professionals showed higher psychoticism levels than females, aligning with prior research. Experienced nurses reported lower personal achievement, hinting at potential motivation challenges for professional growth. Psychoticism predicted high depersonalization and low personal achievement. Neuroticism and psychoticism negatively impacted ICU personnel's mental well-being, reflected in elevated psychopathology scores and burnout status. Psychoticism appears to be the primary factor influencing burnout among the three personality dimensions, particularly affecting intensivists. In contrast, nurses are more influenced by their critical care experience on their mental health status.

Keywords: personality; burnout; nurses; intensivists; intensive care unit; psychopathology

1. Introduction

The term "burnout" was coined by Freudenberger in 1974, who observed declining motivation and commitment among mental health clinic volunteers [1]. Maslach further advanced the concept, creating the widely used Maslach Burnout Inventory (MBI) [2]. According to this framework, burnout syndrome involves emotional exhaustion, physical fatigue, and cognitive weariness due to prolonged uncontrolled work-related stressors [3]. The syndrome comprises three main dimensions: high emotional exhaustion, high depersonalization, and low personal achievement [4]. High emotional exhaustion involves work-related fatigue, marked by feelings of energy depletion, whereas high depersonalization is a defense mechanism, leading to distancing from work through negativism or cynicism. Low personal achievement reflects frustration with work-related achievements, resulting in reduced professional efficiency [4].

Burnout is influenced by enduring personal and environmental stressors, such as major illness, family difficulties, or persistent adversity [5]. In healthcare, burnout syndrome and stress-related disorders are prevalent, impacting various roles like nurses [6,7], emergency room physicians [8], and intensive care unit (ICU) physicians [9,10]. Mental health professionals are also susceptible to high levels of burnout syndrome [11] due to the significant emotional and cognitive stress associated with their profession [12]. Factors associated with physician burnout include age, sex, marital status, personality traits, ICU work experience, work environment, workload, shift work, ethical issues, and end-of-life decision-making [13].

Notably, burnout in physicians is associated with increased risks of major medical errors, reduced patient care quality [14,15], absenteeism, decreased productivity [16–18], and impaired team relationships [19], leading to worsened care quality and higher healthcare costs [3,20]. Nurses often experience burnout due to factors like high workload, value incongruence, low job control, limited decision latitude, poor social climate/support, and insufficient rewards [21]. A common factor across all professions may be the problem of aggression faced by healthcare workers. This aggression, whether it comes from patients or workplace interactions, is considered a precursor to burnout [22–24].

Burnout has emerged as a pervasive issue among healthcare professionals [3]. For example, Woo et al. [25] found that 11.23% of nurses globally have experienced symptoms of burnout. In the field of emergency medicine, healthcare workers exhibit a burnout prevalence rate of 20–60% [26]. Similarly, 40% of mental health professionals have encountered burnout [11], and Rotenstein et al. [27] report that 67% of physicians have demonstrated overall burnout prevalence estimates. In the ICU setting, burnout is reported more prevalently among nurses than physicians [28,29], with direct implications for work, personal functionality, and overall healthcare services [30].

A challenge in current burnout research is the absence of agreed-upon terminology, as demonstrated by the numerous definitions identified, such as in the comprehensive review by Rotenstein et al. [27], covering 182 studies and 109,628 individuals across 45 countries. This lack of consensus leads to widely varying reported prevalence rates, with substantial fluctuations in burnout rates among physicians and within specific subscales [27]. The prevalence of burnout in the ICU setting also shows significant variability [13,31].

Personality traits significantly impact burnout experiences under similar work conditions [32]. Utilizing the dimensions of psychoticism (P), extraversion (E), and neuroticism (N), also known as Eysenck's PEN model [33,34], this study defines personality through these three dimensions [35]. The PEN model posits that these dimensions represent fundamental aspects of an individual's personality, influencing their behavior, cognition, and emotional responses [33,34,36]. Specifically, psychoticism is associated with traits such as disagreeableness, non-conscientiousness, and a propensity for risk-taking. Extraversion encompasses characteristics like sociability, assertiveness, positive emotions, and impulsivity, while neuroticism involves traits such as anxiety, depression, and self-doubt. Furthermore, these personality dimensions—P, E, and N—are considered orthogonal [37], indicating no correlation between them, thus contributing to a comprehensive understanding of various facets of an individual's personality [36].

Neuroticism and lower extraversion are commonly associated with elevated burnout levels among nurses and physicians [29,38–43]. However, there is a notable scarcity of studies comparing personality traits between nurses and physicians [44], particularly within the ICU environment. Understanding such distinctions could have far-reaching implications for team dynamics, patient care, workplace satisfaction, and healthcare system improvement.

Personality differences are observed among rural and urban residents, with environmental factors influencing personality structure and exacerbating feelings of anxiety and depression [45,46]. Urban characteristics, such as exposure to heavy metals, pesticides, bisphenol A (BPA), noise pollution, and poor air quality, are linked to mental health conditions [47–52]. In Greek metropolitan areas like Athens and Thessaloniki, high population density and limited green spaces pose challenges [53]. Despite these, specialized hospitals in these regions serve wider areas in southern and northern Greece. The lower nurse-to-ICU bed ratio in metropolitan hospitals during COVID-19 [54] suggests an added psychological burden on ICU personnel, raising questions about the mental impact on healthcare workers in large urban areas compared to smaller cities.

Aim of the Study

This study delves into the intricate connections among socio-demographics, personality traits, psychopathology, and burnout in ICU personnel. Using a moderated mediation model, it explores the nuanced interplay involving critical care experience, personality dimensions, burnout, profession, and hospital location. Critical care experience serves as the independent variable, with personality dimensions mediating the relationship between experience and burnout. Additionally, the nurse or intensivist profession and the urban status of the hospital act as moderators, examining variations based on professional role and urban size. This design allows for assessing both direct and mediated effects as well as investigating whether the mediation process varies with moderator variables. In essence, we tested the moderated mediation model illustrated in Figure 1.

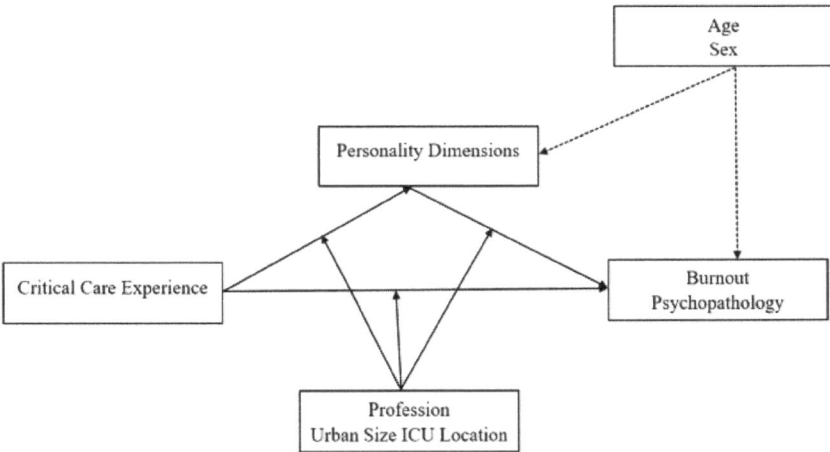

Figure 1. Theoretical moderated mediation model. Notes: Personality dimensions are hypothesized to mediate the relationship between critical care experience and burnout/psychopathology. In contrast, profession, and urban size of ICU location (and potentially age and sex) are hypothesized to moderate the relationships within the model.

Among other inquiries, the model addresses the following research questions:
- How do personality dimensions differentiate as age increase?
- How do personality traits vary between male and female ICU personnel?
- What is the relationship between critical care experience, burnout, and psychopathology?
- Does the relationship between critical care experience, burnout, and psychopathology vary depending on the profession or the urban size of the ICU location?
- How do personality dimensions and profession interact in predicting burnout?
- Does the effect of critical care experience on burnout and psychopathology vary between nurses and intensivists or between ICU location in small and large cities?

Understanding these connections is vital for theoretical advancement and targeted interventions to improve the well-being of ICU personnel. This research has the potential to contribute to tailored support systems, addressing the unique needs of intensivists and nurses in high-stress environments.

2. Methods

2.1. Participants and Study Design

This study involved a cross-sectional investigation conducted with a sample of 573 respondents drawn from 31 ICUs in 10 cities across Greece. The sampling process took place between December 2021 and June 2022. Out of the total 573 ICU personnel, 23 individuals were excluded from subsequent analysis as they did not fit the roles of nurses or physicians. Additionally, from the remaining 550 participants, 47 were identified with at least one missing value in the required demographic or professional characteristics, leading to their exclusion from further analysis. Consequently, the results presented in this study are based on data obtained from the remaining 503 respondents, comprising 155 intensivists and 348 nurses.

2.2. Measurements

The participants were asked to anonymously complete a sociodemographic questionnaire, which encompassed necessary personal and professional information. Additionally, they were required to fill out the adapted to Greek-language versions of the Maslach Burnout Inventory (MBI) [55], the Eysenck Personality Questionnaire (EPQ) [56], and the Symptom Checklist 90 (SCL-90) [57].

The MBI, developed by Maslach and Jackson [2], assesses burnout through 22 items grouped into three subscales: emotional exhaustion, depersonalization, and personal achievement. Respondents rate each item on a 7-point Likert scale ranging from 'never' (0) to 'daily' (6). The scale has been translated into Greek and has shown satisfactory validity and reliability [55]. In this study, we used the established thresholds on the three subscales, based on the adapted Greek version by Zis et al. [58]. Specifically, burnout was identified for scores ≥ 34 in emotional exhaustion, ≥ 13 in depersonalization, and ≤ 29 in personal achievement.

The EPQ, developed by Eysenck and Eysenck [35], assesses personality traits using a 90-item questionnaire. It measures three primary dimensions: extraversion, neuroticism, and psychoticism. Respondents rate each item on a binary scale (yes/no response). The scale has been translated into Greek and has shown satisfactory validity and reliability [56].

The SCL-90, developed by Derogatis [59], assesses a wide range of psychological symptoms. It comprises 90 questions across 9 subscales, namely somatization, obsessive-compulsive, interpersonal sensitivity, depression, anxiety, hostility, phobic anxiety, paranoid ideation, and psychoticism. Participants rate items on a 5-point Likert scale ranging from 0 (not at all) to 4 (extremely) based on distress level. Additionally, three global indices (global severity index [GSI], positive symptom distress index [PSDI], and positive symptom total [PST]) summarize psychological distress. The scale has been translated into Greek and validated for criterion and convergent validity [57]. This study reports data only for the GSI index, a measure that reflects the overall psychopathology. A higher GSI score indicates higher levels of psychological distress.

Participants provided verbal informed consent prior to their involvement in the study, and ethical approval was granted by the Ethics Committee of the University Hospital of Ioannina (protocol code 3263, dated 1 February 2019). Participants were also assigned unique identifiers to anonymize their data, and only authorized researchers had access to the raw data.

2.3. Statistical Analysis

Initial data analysis involved summarizing measures of central tendency and dispersion, with means and standard deviations reported for continuous variables and proportions for categorical ones. To compare groups, we employed independent samples t-tests, chi-squared tests of independence, and one-way ANOVA. To evaluate the internal consistency and reliability of the utilized scales—namely, the MBI, the EPQ, and the SCL-90—Cronbach's alpha analysis was conducted [60]. Additionally, a Pearson correlation analysis was executed to examine the correlation matrix, encompassing age, personality traits, burnout, and psychopathology.

To evaluate the theoretical model, a moderated mediation approach was employed, wherein the relationship between critical care experience and burnout was mediated by three personality dimensions, while profession moderated this relationship (Figure 1). Model 76 of the PROCESS function for R, developed by Hayes [61], was utilized four times: once for each facet of burnout (i.e., emotional exhaustion, depersonalization, and personal achievement) [58] and once for the psychopathology, as indicated by the GSI [57]. This model was chosen for its robust capabilities in handling moderated mediation models [61].

Furthermore, we categorized critical care experience into three groups: less than 5 years, 5–10 years, and more than 10 years. Each group was compared to the preceding group using a sequential coding scheme [61]. This approach facilitated the comparison of successive levels of experience and enabled a nuanced exploration of the progressive nature of phenomena within the ICU setting. In both the moderation analysis of personality dimensions and the moderation analysis of burnout and psychopathology, main effects and interaction effects were examined. Bootstrap analysis was conducted to evaluate the indirect effects of the theoretical model. Unstandardized coefficients (B) and 95% confidence intervals were reported. Additionally, we reported the R^2 for each model to assess the proportion of variance explained. Significant interaction effects were graphically illustrated. The statistical analysis was conducted under the guidance of a statistician to ensure accuracy and rigor in the interpretation of results.

A two-sided alpha level of 0.05 was set for determining statistical significance. All data were analyzed using the R (version 4.2.3) statistical language [62] equipped with the PROCESS function [61].

3. Results

3.1. Sample Demographics

Among the 503 respondents, nurses were notably younger (39.6 ± 7.8 vs. 45.7 ± 8.1, $t(501) = 7.935$, $p < 0.001$), more likely to be female (74.4% vs. 51.6%, $\chi^2(1) = 25.397$, $p < 0.001$), and had less experience in the ICU environment compared to the intensivists ($\chi^2(2) = 20.579$, $p < 0.001$).

3.2. Personality, Burnout, and Psychopathology Profiles

The psychometric scales used in this study demonstrated acceptable internal reliability, as evidenced by the examination of Cronbach's alpha (a) coefficient (Table 1) [60]. The three personality traits were weakly correlated between them, confirming the assumed orthogonality [36,37]. Additionally, a notable positive correlation was reported between emotional exhaustion and depersonalization.

Table 1. Correlation between personality traits and burnout facets of the examined sample.

		a	Personality Traits			Burnout Facets		
			Extraversion	Neuroticism	Psychoticism	Emotional Exhaustion	Depersonalization	Personal Achievement
Personality Traits	Extraversion	0.871						
	Neuroticism	0.951	−0.127 **					
	Psychoticism	0.907	−0.180 **	0.225 **				
Burnout facets	Emotional exhaustion	0.839	−0.131 **	0.370 **	0.133 **			
	Depersonalization	0.767	−0.078	0.297 **	0.277 **	0.624 **		
	Personal achievement	0.828	0.345 **	−0.167 **	−0.349 **	−0.045	−0.128 **	
Global severity index (GSI)		0.99	−0.168 **	0.476 **	0.474 **	0.512 **	0.431 **	−0.197 **

Notes: a = Cronbach's alpha, ** correlation significant at 0.01 level.

Table 2 presents the descriptive statistics of personality traits, burnout scores, and psychopathology for the total sample as well as stratified by profession, sex, critical care experience, and urban size of ICU location.

Table 2. Personality, burnout, and psychopathology of the examined sample.

Scale	Total (N = 503)	Profession		Sex		Critical Care Experience			Urban Size of ICU Location	
		Intensivist (n = 155)	Nurse (n = 348)	Male (n = 164)	Female (n = 339)	<5 Years (n = 166)	5–10 Years (n = 105)	10–15 Years (n = 232)	Metropolitan (n = 309)	Other (n = 194)
Age	41.5 (8.4)	45.7 (8.1)	39.6 (7.8)	43.0 (8.8)	41.0 (8.1)	35 (6.4)	42 (7.0)	46 (7.1)	41.6 (8.5)	41.4 (8.2)
Personality traits										
Psychoticism	5.8 (3.9)	4.5 (3.2)	6.3 (4.0)	6.3 (4.3)	5.5 (3.7)	4.9 (3.1)	6.6 (4.5)	5.9 (4.0)	5.8 (4)	5.7 (3.8)
Extraversion	12.2 (4.3)	12.1 (4.26)	12.2 (4.3)	12.1 (4.2)	12.2 (4.3)	13.2 (4.2)	12.0 (4.2)	11.0 (4.2)	12.2 (4.2)	12.1 (4.4)
Neuroticism	10.7 (4.5)	9.85 (4.62)	11.1 (4.4)	10.2 (4.8)	10.9 (4.4)	9.6 (4.3)	11.0 (4.7)	11.0 (4.4)	10.5 (4.3)	10.9 (4.9)
Burnout facets										
Emotional exhaustion	25.6 (11.1)	24.4 (10.8)	26.2 (11.2)	24.8 (11.6)	26 (10.8)	23.7 (10.3)	25.0 (11.0)	27.0 (11.0)	26 (11.2)	25 (10.9)
Depersonalization	10.4 (6.6)	10.1 (7.0)	10.6 (6.4)	10.8 (7.0)	10.3 (6.4)	9.5 (6.3)	10.0 (6.5)	11.0 (6.7)	10.8 (6.6)	9.9 (6.6)
Personal achievement	31.2 (8.7)	33.7 (7.1)	30.1 (9.1)	32.2 (8.4)	30.7 (8.8)	32.5 (7.7)	30.0 (10.0)	31.0 (8.7)	31.7 (8.4)	30.5 (9.1)
Global severity index (GSI)	0.89 (0.72)	0.72 (0.57)	0.96 (0.77)	0.84 (0.81)	0.91 (0.67)	0.71 (0.60)	1.1 (0.87)	0.93 (0.70)	0.92 (0.73)	0.85 (0.70)

Notes: N = total sample size (intensivists and nurses), n = sample size per group, ICU = intensive care unit. Means and standard deviations are presented.

As shown in Table 3, a total of 129 participants, 38 intensivists and 91 nurses, were classified as experiencing high emotional exhaustion. Additionally, 195 participants, 43 intensivists and 152 nurses, were identified as having low personal achievement. Furthermore, 188 participants, 59 intensivists and 129 nurses, were categorized as experiencing high levels of depersonalization (Table 3).

Table 3. Concurrence among burnout facets of the examined sample.

Emotional Exhaustion	Depersonalization	Personal Achievement		
		Low (≤29)	Moderate (30–38)	High (≥39)
Low (≤16)	Low (≤4)	20 (12/8) [1]	16 (5/11)	9 (4/5)
	Moderate (5–12)	13 (7/6)	14 (7/7)	27 (2/25)
	High (≥13)	5 (2/3)	1 (0/1)	0 (0/0)
Moderate (17–33)	Low (≤4)	21 (8/13)	25 (11/14)	10 (2/8)
	Moderate (5–12)	20 (9/11)	52 (11/41)	48 (8/40)
	High (≥13)	13 (2/11)	34 (13/21)	46 (14/32)
High (≥34)	Low (≤4)	2 (1/1)	2 (1/1)	0 (0/0)
	Moderate (5–12)	2 (1/1)	11 (4/7)	23 (3/20)
	High (≥13)	19 (5/14)	38 (13/25)	32 (10/22)

Notes: [1] frequencies of total sample (frequencies of intensivists/frequencies of nurses).

The profession in the ICU was not related with the status of a high emotional exhaustion ($c2(1) = 0.15$, $p = 0.699$) and high depersonalization ($c2(1) = 0.045$, $p = 0.831$), while it was more probable for nurses to report a low personal achievement score ($c2(1) = 11.473$, $p = 0.001$). The GSI was significantly correlated with emotional exhaustion and depersonalization scores and exhibited a negative correlation with the personal achievement score. Specifically, the GSI was significantly higher among the respondents characterized as individuals experiencing high emotional exhaustion (1.37 vs. 0.72, $t(501) = 9.508$,

$p < 0.001$) as well as among those characterized as individuals with high depersonalization (1.23 vs. 0.68, t (501) = 8.828, $p < 0.001$) or low personal achievement (1.05 vs. 0.79, t (501) = 4.098, $p < 0.001$).

3.3. Moderation Analysis of Personality Dimensions

The effect of demographics and the experience in the ICU environment on personality dimensions are presented in Table 4. Age was not found to have a significant effect on the three personality dimensions. Instead, a sex-based disparity was reported, with male healthcare professionals demonstrating markedly elevated levels of psychoticism compared to their female counterparts (M = 6.3 vs. M = 5.5, $p < 0.001$). A noteworthy main effect of profession on neuroticism emerged, indicating that nurses exhibited higher levels of neuroticism in comparison to intensivists (M = 11.1 vs. M = 9.9, $p = 0.038$).

Table 4. Moderation analysis of personality dimensions of the examined sample.

	Neuroticism [1]				Psychoticism [2]				Extraversion [3]			
	B	p	95% C.I. Lower	95% C.I. Upper	B	p	95% C.I. Lower	95% C.I. Upper	B	p	95% C.I. Lower	95% C.I. Upper
Constant	5.283	0.028	0.562	10.00	5.157	0.009	1.275	9.039	11.07	0.000	6.600	15.55
					Critical Care Experience							
D_1: 5–10 vs. <5	1.364	0.700	−5.598	8.326	−5.543	0.058	−11.27	0.180	0.522	0.877	−6.073	7.116
D_2: 10–15 vs. 5–10	4.231	0.194	−2.155	10.62	1.642	0.539	−3.608	6.892	2.152	0.485	−3.896	8.201
Profession	**1.693**	**0.038**	**0.091**	**3.294**	−0.289	0.666	−1.606	1.027	**1.721**	**0.026**	**0.204**	**3.238**
					Critical Care Experience × Profession							
D_1 × Profess.	−0.311	0.824	−3.065	2.442	**3.883**	**0.001**	**1.620**	**6.147**	−1.246	0.348	−3.855	1.362
D_2 × Profess.	−0.001	0.999	−2.556	2.554	−0.444	0.678	−2.545	1.656	−2.074	0.093	−4.494	0.346
Urban size of ICU Location	0.771	0.287	−0.651	2.194	0.370	0.534	−0.799	1.540	−0.325	0.636	−1.672	1.022
					Critical Care Experience × Uban Size of ICU Location							
D_1 × Urban Size of ICU Location	0.288	0.808	−2.040	2.615	0.424	0.663	−1.489	2.337	0.295	0.793	−1.909	2.499
D_2 × Urban Size of ICU Location	**−2.216**	**0.046**	**−4.392**	**−0.040**	−0.515	0.572	−2.304	1.273	0.406	0.699	−1.655	2.467
Age	0.004	0.907	−0.057	0.064	−0.027	0.289	−0.076	0.023	−0.006	0.824	−0.064	0.051
Sex	−0.199	0.647	−1.054	0.655	**1.421**	**0.000**	**0.719**	**2.123**	−0.246	0.550	−1.055	0.563

Notes: D = duration of critical care experience based on years of experience, B = unstandardized estimates, p = p-value, C.I. = confidence interval, ICU = intensive care unit, R^2 = R-squared measure that represents the proportion of the variance in the dependent variable, significant differences are marked with bold, [1] $R^2 = 0.067$, $F (10, 492) = 3.531$, $p < 0.001$. [2] $R^2 = 0.147$, $F (10, 492) = 8.491$, $p < 0.001$. [3] $R^2 = 0.062$, $F (10,492) = 3.342$, $p < 0.001$.

Furthermore, our analysis showed some significant interaction effects (Table 2), which are further illustrated in Figure 2, Panel A–C. A noteworthy interaction between critical care experience and urban size of the ICU location concerning neuroticism was observed, suggesting that ICU personnel in minor cities tend to report higher levels of neuroticism across all experience levels than those in metropolitan cities, with the greatest difference seen in the group with more than 10 years of experience (Figure 2, Panel A). Additionally, the analysis revealed a significant interaction between critical care experience and profession regarding psychoticism and extraversion. Specifically, as experience in the ICU increases, nurses exhibited higher levels of psychoticism and lower levels of extraversion (Figure 2, Panel B,C).

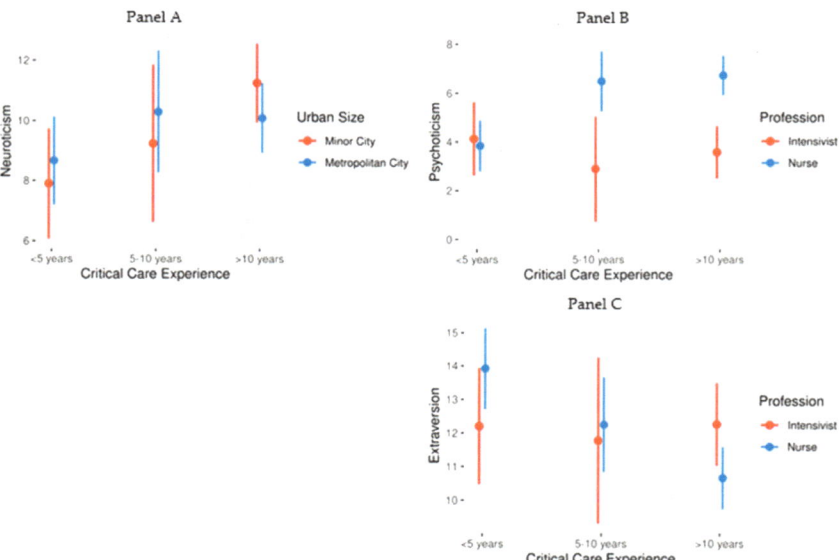

Figure 2. Interaction effects of critical care experience, urban size of ICU location, and profession on the personality traits in the context of the examined model. Notes: The length of critical care experience was categorized into three groups: less than 5 years, 5–10 years, and more than 10 years. (**Panel A**) Differences in neuroticism were assessed across these groups by the urban size of ICU location categorized as 'minor city' and 'metropolitan city'. Differences in psychoticism (**Panel B**) and extraversion (**Panel C**) were assessed across these groups by the profession categorized as 'intensivist' and 'nurse'. Each dot represents the mean score for the respective group, while the error bars signify 95% confidence intervals.

3.4. Moderation Analysis of Burnout Facets and Psychopathology

The analysis uncovered notable associations between age and various dimensions of psychological well-being among the participants (Table 5). Specifically, a significant positive effect emerged between age and the likelihood of experiencing high emotional exhaustion (B = 0.037, p = 0.027), signifying a 1.4 times increase in the odds of high emotional exhaustion for each additional decade in the respondents' age. Conversely, a negative relationship was identified between age and the likelihood of experiencing low personal accomplishment (B = −0.050, p = 0.004), suggesting a 0.6 times decrease in the odds of low personal accomplishment for each additional decade in the respondents' age. Additionally, a noteworthy positive association was observed between age and the GSI (B = 0.009, p = 0.020), indicating a 0.09 increase in the GSI score for each additional decade in the respondents' age. Furthermore, the personality trait of neuroticism (B = 0.082, p = 0.011) was identified as significant regressor of the GSI score, emphasizing its meaningful contribution to the overall psychological well-being of the participants (Table 5).

Table 5. Moderation analysis of burnout and psychopathology of the examined sample.

	High Emotional Exhaustion [1]				High Depersonalization [2]				Low Personal Achievement [3]				Global Severity Index (GSI) [4]			
	B	p	95% C.I. Lower	95% C.I. Upper	B	p	95% C.I. Lower	95% C.I. Upper	B	p	95% C.I. Lower	95% C.I. Upper	B	p	95% C.I. Lower	95% C.I. Upper
Constant	−0.571	0.840	−6.126	4.984	−2.857	0.277	−8.006	2.292	0.130	0.962	−5.190	5.451	−0.367	0.578	−1.662	0.929
								Socio-demographics								
Age	**0.037**	**0.027**	**0.004**	**0.071**	0.017	0.265	−0.013	0.047	**−0.050**	**0.004**	**−0.084**	**−0.015**	**0.009**	**0.020**	**0.001**	**0.017**
Sex	0.135	0.588	−0.353	0.623	0.018	0.937	−0.422	0.458	−0.449	0.070	−0.934	0.037	−0.070	0.230	−0.183	0.044
								Critical Care Experience								
D$_1$: 5–10 vs. <5	−1.365	0.532	−5.644	2.914	−2.395	0.249	−6.470	1.681	0.434	0.832	−3.565	4.432	−0.174	0.712	−1.102	0.753
D$_2$: 10–15 vs. 5–10	0.938	0.626	−2.835	4.712	2.438	0.194	−1.244	6.119	−4.318	0.025	−8.092	−0.545	−0.113	0.790	−0.950	0.723
D$_1$ × Profession	−0.904	0.431	−3.153	1.345	0.261	0.804	−1.800	2.322	0.944	0.387	−1.196	3.085	0.132	0.614	−0.381	0.645
D$_2$ × Profession	−0.138	0.869	−1.772	1.496	0.736	0.399	−0.975	2.448	−0.031	0.970	−1.619	1.558	−0.005	0.976	−0.371	0.360
Urban Size of ICU Location	0.485	0.514	−0.972	1.942	−1.356	0.092	−2.934	0.222	**1.967**	**0.012**	**0.433**	**3.501**	0.062	0.714	−0.272	0.397
D$_1$ × Urban Size of ICU Location	−1.472	0.172	−3.585	0.642	−0.225	0.813	−2.091	1.641	0.060	0.950	−1.842	1.963	−0.178	0.468	−0.658	0.303
D$_2$ × Urban Size of ICU Location	0.708	0.355	−0.791	2.208	0.554	0.368	−0.652	1.760	−0.160	0.803	−1.418	1.098	0.151	0.338	−0.159	0.462
D$_3$ × Urban Size of ICU Location	−0.664	0.329	−1.998	0.669	0.238	0.672	−0.863	1.339	0.674	0.260	−0.499	1.846	−0.068	0.639	−0.355	0.218
								Personality Traits								
P	0.229	0.189	−0.113	0.571	**0.455**	**0.014**	**0.092**	**0.818**	**0.488**	**0.014**	**0.098**	**0.877**	0.029	0.502	−0.056	0.114
E	−0.234	0.105	−0.518	0.049	−0.207	0.121	−0.470	0.055	−0.224	0.148	−0.528	0.080	−0.019	0.578	−0.085	0.048
N	−0.039	0.782	−0.315	0.237	0.168	0.191	−0.084	0.421	**0.327**	**0.033**	**0.026**	**0.627**	**0.082**	**0.011**	**0.019**	**0.145**
P × Profession	−0.099	0.147	−0.233	0.035	**−0.233**	**0.003**	**−0.388**	**−0.077**	**−0.182**	**0.029**	**−0.346**	**−0.019**	−0.011	0.529	−0.045	0.023
E × Profession	0.060	0.311	−0.056	0.175	0.098	0.072	−0.009	0.205	0.009	0.885	−0.113	0.131	−0.001	0.928	−0.028	0.026
N × Profession	0.066	0.237	−0.044	0.176	−0.012	0.814	−0.113	0.088	−0.086	0.162	−0.206	0.034	−0.001	0.911	−0.027	0.024
P × Urban Size of ICU Location	−0.019	0.759	−0.141	0.103	0.039	0.487	−0.071	0.150	0.001	0.982	−0.120	0.123	**0.036**	**0.017**	**0.006**	**0.065**
E × Urban Size of ICU Location	0.087	0.112	−0.021	0.195	0.022	0.658	−0.075	0.119	0.045	0.422	−0.064	0.154	0.009	0.476	−0.016	0.034
N × Urban Size of ICU Location	0.037	0.504	−0.071	0.145	−0.044	0.368	−0.139	0.051	−0.088	0.098	−0.193	0.016	−0.012	0.354	−0.036	0.013

Notes: D = duration of critical care experience based on years of experience, D$_1$: 5–10 vs. <5, D$_2$: 10–15 vs. 5–10, ICU = intensive care unit, R^2 = R-squared measure that represents the proportion of the variance in the dependent variable, P = psychoticism, E = extraversion, N = neuroticism, significant differences are marked with bold, [1] $R^2 = 0.156$, $c2(19) = 56.298$, $p < 0.001$. [2] $R^2 = 0.157$, $c2(19) = 61.324$, $p < 0.001$. [3] $R^2 = 0.321$, $c2(19) = 135.995$, $p < 0.001$. [4] $R^2 = 0.398$, F (19, 483) = 16.837, $p < 0.001$.

Additionally, the analysis revealed significant interaction effects (Table 5) between psychoticism, critical care experience, profession, and the urban size of the ICU location, which are further illustrated in Figure 3, Panel A–D. Notably, with an increasing duration of critical care experience, nurses tended to report lower personal achievement scores, whereas intensivists showed an opposite trend (Figure 3, Panel A). Moreover, the relationship between psychoticism and psychopathology, as measured by the GSI, varied in strength depending on the urban size of the ICU location. Specifically, ICU personnel in larger metropolitan areas exhibited a more robust relationship between psychoticism and GSI scores than those in smaller urban settings (Figure 3, Panel B). Lastly, there was a significant association between psychoticism and both low personal achievement and high depersonalization scores. This relationship was particularly strong among intensivists when compared to nurses (Figure 3, Panel C,D).

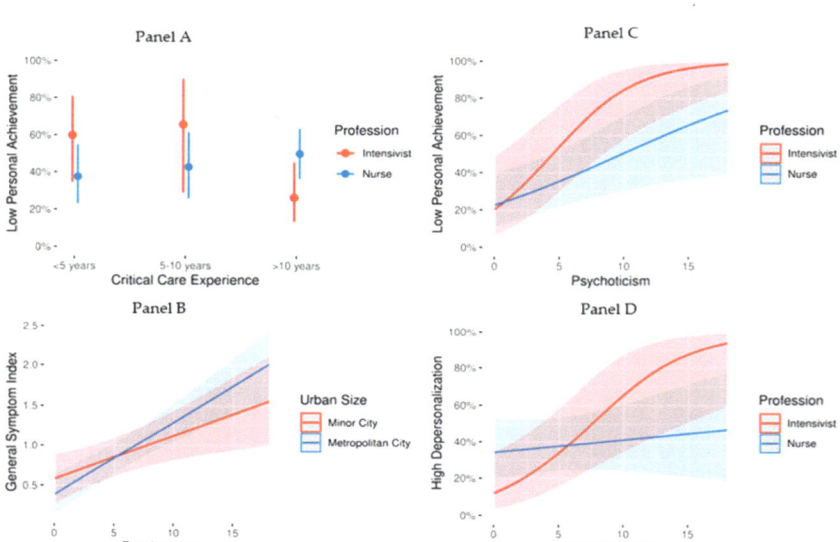

Figure 3. Interaction effects of critical care experience, profession, and urban size of ICU location on the probability of burnout symptoms and psychopathology in the context of the examined model. Notes: (**Panel A**) The probability of low personal achievement across different levels of critical care experience for the two professions. Each dot represents the mean score for the respective group, while the error bars signify 95% confidence intervals. (**Panel B**) The psychopathology scores against levels of psychoticism for individuals in metropolitan versus minor cities. The shaded areas around the lines represent 95% confidence intervals, while the lines show that as psychoticism increased, so did the psychopathology score, with a stronger effect seen in metropolitan areas. (**Panel C**) The relationship between the personality trait of psychoticism and the probability of low personal achievement for intensivists and nurses. The shaded areas around the lines represent 95% confidence intervals. The upward trend for both lines suggests that as psychoticism increased, the likelihood of low personal achievement also increased, with a steeper slope for intensivists than for nurses. (**Panel D**) The probability of experiencing high depersonalization against the level of psychoticism for intensivists and nurses. The shaded areas around the lines represent 95% confidence intervals. The trend indicates that higher levels of psychoticism were associated with a higher probability of experiencing high depersonalization. The difference in slopes between the two professions suggests that the effect of psychoticism on depersonalization was more pronounced in intensivists.

3.5. Indirect Effects

In the context of the examined model, the bootstrap analysis showed that personality dimensions did not have a significant indirect effect on the relationship between critical care experience and both psychopathology and burnout.

4. Discussion

4.1. Personality Dimensions

The three personality traits exhibited weak correlations (Pearson's r < 0.3), affirming the assumed orthogonality between psychoticism, extraversion, and neuroticism [36,37,63,64]. The observation that male healthcare professionals manifested notably elevated levels of psychoticism in comparison to their female counterparts substantiates the hypothesized association with psychoticism. In contrast, the inconclusive sex differences reported for extraversion align with analogous evidence in the literature [65,66], irrespective of the specific measurement instrument employed [36,67].

The extant literature lacks consensus regarding whether nurses lean towards extroversion or introversion, with several reports suggesting tendencies in either direction [44]. Particularly among ICU nurses, their personality traits were characterized by higher scores on dominance, rebelliousness, and self-sufficiency, coupled with lower scores on emotional sensitivity and imagination compared to nurses from other departments [68,69], predominantly indicative of elevated psychoticism. The observation that, with increasing experience in the ICU, nurses exhibit higher levels of psychoticism and diminished levels of extraversion further elucidates the reported relations. This suggests that in the high-pressure environment of an ICU, nurses may develop heightened psychoticism and reduced extraversion as adaptive coping mechanisms in response to stress and the demanding nature of their roles [70].

This phenomenon may be linked to challenges faced by nurses in establishing effective communication with patients who often experience objective communication difficulties [71,72] and frequently undergo negative emotional reactions such as frustration, stress, anxiety, and depression [73,74]. Given that effective human-level interaction forms the cornerstone of a positive working environment for nurses, it is plausible to posit that persistent challenges in communication may predispose nurses to heightened feelings of anxiety, depression, self-doubt, and other negative emotions, contributing to an elevated psychoticism score. In this context, previous assertions highlighting inferior personality factors linked to communication skills in ICU nurses compared to hospitalization unit nurses [75] should not be attributed to systematic personality variance among nurses. Instead, it is crucial to recognize that these disparities may originate from substantial barriers to effective communication [76].

Contrastingly, as experience in the ICU increases, intensivists experience heightened neuroticism, indicating an increased sense of responsibility and concern for patient outcomes. However, this also implies a higher emotional and psychosomatic toll in managing critically ill patients over time in the ICU. Given that elevated neuroticism is typically associated with an increased risk of mental illness [77] and, on average, poorer outcomes in terms of health and relationship satisfaction [78,79], a necessity emerges for a more palliative approach for long-term ICU doctors.

4.2. Burnout and Psychopathology

No overall significant differences were observed between nurses and intensivists regarding burnout status, aligning with prior research findings [80,81]. However, this stands in contrast to other studies [28,29]. This discrepancy in findings might be attributable to the specific samples and settings of the various studies. In relation to personal achievement, an inverse relationship between age and the likelihood of a low score status was identified, implying that with increasing age and experience, healthcare professionals acquire enhanced coping mechanisms for the emotional and physical stressors inherent in ICU settings [82]. However, an intriguing dynamic is suggested by the discovery that intensivists with lower

ICU experience exhibit a higher probability of reporting low personal achievement compared to ICU nurses with equivalent experience. This pattern is reversed among intensivists and nurses with greater ICU experience. The origin of this phenomenon remains uncertain but may be attributed to distinct professional obligations in an ICU setting, with intensivists typically assuming more leadership and decision-making responsibilities than nurses [83]. Consequently, lower-experience intensivists may find these responsibilities overwhelming early in their careers, resulting in a sense of lower personal achievement. Nevertheless, with accumulated experience, they may become more adept at managing complex cases, leading to an improved sense of accomplishment. Conversely, experienced nurses may perceive stagnation in their careers, with limited opportunities for advancement, autonomy, or professional growth. The absence of well-defined career paths can foster a sense of being trapped in their current position, potentially leading to increased job stress and a diminished sense of accomplishment [84–86].

Interestingly, a positive correlation was found between age and personal achievement among ICU personnel, with increasing age associated with a lower likelihood of reporting low personal accomplishment. This trend suggests that with advancing age, there is a discernible decrease in reporting low levels of personal accomplishment, indicating that older ICU personnel may perceive their professional achievements more positively. This can largely be attributed to the cumulative effect of accrued experience over time in relation to job satisfaction [87], which ostensibly contributes to a more favorable self-assessment of accomplishments in the challenging ICU environment. Therefore, the career trajectory of healthcare professionals in such settings might be characterized by a gradual and steady increase in personal accomplishment, underpinned by the development of adaptive skills and psychological resilience.

In contrast, there was a significant negative correlation between age and emotional exhaustion and psychopathology, confirming a general trend towards an increased feeling of emotional exhaustion in older ICU personnel, as reported in various studies [88–90]. This finding is another manifestation of the mental burden derived from the recent health crisis, resulting in a significant psychological toll and high burnout rates in the global healthcare community [81,91,92], particularly among Greek healthcare professionals [93–96]. Accordingly, the commonly reported notion that accumulated work experience and resulting physical and mental fatigue contribute to a higher overall psychopathology is confirmed [92,97–99].

The adverse implications of high neuroticism or high psychoticism scores are further evident in their direct effects on the psychopathology, aligning with prior reports [77,100,101]. Additionally, the added effect of stressors related to urban living, such as long commutes and a high cost of living, is reflected in the stronger relationship of personality traits like psychoticism with general psychopathology symptoms. This amplification could be particularly pronounced in high-stress healthcare settings, where the additional urban stressors can intensify the psychological impact of already demanding jobs. Studies have shown that environmental factors like urban living conditions can significantly affect mental health, potentially exacerbating underlying personality traits [102,103]. Additionally, the role of organizational culture in hospitals, especially in metropolitan areas, is critical. A less supportive work environment and limited mental health resources can leave ICU personnel, particularly those with higher psychoticism scores, more vulnerable to psychological distress and less equipped to cope effectively. The importance of organizational support in mitigating the impact of stress on mental health has been emphasized in various studies [104–107].

Secondly, the personality dimension of psychoticism was highlighted as an important predictor of the probability of high depersonalization and low personal achievement scores, confirming previous reports [38,108]. Specifically, feelings within the psychotic spectrum, such as irritability and quick-tempered reactions, a tendency to be suspicious of others' motives or actions, feelings of restlessness, and general inner tension are valid signs of less psychological resilience and are significantly associated with a higher likelihood of perceiving incompetence, unsuccessful outcomes in their work, and a cynical behavior toward colleagues and patients [109]. Further, the association between psychoticism and lower personal achievement and higher depersonalization may be more pronounced among intensivists due to the increased responsibility and decisional burden associated with their roles, documented to impact decreased job satisfaction and emotional and psychological burnout [110,111]. Specifically, psychoticism, with its resilience traits, might influence how intensivists cope with the emotional challenges, potentially exacerbating the negative outcomes observed. Furthermore, the hierarchical nature of healthcare settings, combined with the intense and challenging work environment of the ICU, may amplify the association between psychoticism and adverse outcomes among intensivists. Nurses, although impacted, might not experience the same level of intensity and pressure in their roles.

Finally, this study found that personality traits do not significantly influence the relationship between critical care experience, psychopathology, and burnout. Essentially, the direct effects of critical care experience on both psychopathology and burnout are substantial enough to explain their relationships without the need to consider personality traits as an explanatory factor. This suggests that the impact of critical care experience on psychopathology and burnout occurs independently of an individual's personality traits.

5. Conclusions

This study explored the relationships between personality traits, burnout, and psychopathology among ICU personnel, considering the moderating effect of experience and workplace setting. Among ICU nurses, increasing experience was correlated with higher psychoticism and lower extraversion, potentially as a coping mechanism for communication difficulties. Intensivists with lower ICU experience reported higher burnout. Psychoticism and neuroticism had direct effects on psychopathology, with stronger relations in metropolitan areas. Psychoticism predicted high depersonalization and low personal achievement, particularly among intensivists, indicating potential implications for coping with emotional challenges and adverse outcomes in high-pressure healthcare settings.

The findings underscore the need for a holistic understanding of the psychosocial dynamics within ICU settings, acknowledging the impact of communication challenges and the evolving responsibilities of healthcare roles. It is important to note that the repercussions of high levels of burnout and psychopathology among ICU personnel are significant, impacting both the healthcare professionals themselves [3,6,112] and the quality of patient care [113]. Research indicates that healthcare personnel experiencing burnout are associated with adverse patient outcomes. This includes diminished patient safety [114,115], increased standardized mortality ratios, and prolonged hospitalization durations [116]. Additionally, there is a correlation between healthcare worker burnout and reduced patient satisfaction [117] as well as an increased incidence of medical errors and malpractice [14,15,113].

Our study, therefore, lays a foundation for future explorations into strategic interventions aimed at establishing specialized training programs and robust support frameworks within the ICU. These programs and support systems are envisioned to offer both emotional and professional assistance to ICU personnel, thereby enhancing their ability to effectively manage the intense stress characteristic of the ICU and urban environment. Such proactive measures are crucial for maintaining the mental well-being and professional efficacy of ICU personnel.

Limitations

It is imperative to acknowledge certain limitations in the interpretation and generalization of this study's findings. Primarily, our results are based on a sample of ICU personnel from Greece, limiting generalizability beyond populations with similar cultural backgrounds, such as Mediterranean countries, cautioning against universal application to regions with distinct social structures. To enhance generalizability, future studies should include ICU personnel from various regions and cultural backgrounds. Conducting longitudinal research, as opposed to the cross-sectional approach used in this study, could offer insights into how these relationships evolve over time, particularly how personality traits interact with burnout and psychopathology in the long run. Additionally, comparing ICU personnel in urban versus rural settings, or in different healthcare systems, might reveal how environmental and systemic factors influence these relationships.

Secondly, the moderated mediation model employed in this research focused on the relationship between critical care experience, personality traits, burnout, and psychopathology. As such, the results are constrained by the specific pathways and variables within this model. While our study provides valuable insights into these particular associations, it does not capture the entirety of the complex interactions between personality dimensions and psychopathology. Other unexplored variables and pathways may exist, and the extent to which our findings can be extrapolated to a broader context may be limited. Exploring factors such as workplace environment, support systems, and personal life stressors could provide a more comprehensive understanding of the dynamics at play. Therefore, future research should consider additional factors and pathways to gain a more comprehensive understanding of the complex relationship between personality traits, burnout, and psychopathology in the context of ICU personnel. Finally, qualitative studies, such as interviews or focus groups, could provide deeper insights into the personal experiences and perspectives of ICU personnel, which might be missed in quantitative models.

Author Contributions: Conceptualization, V.K., M.G. and V.P.; methodology, V.K., G.P. and M.G.; software, M.G., D.T. and E.D.; validation, V.K., G.P. and D.T.; investigation, V.P.; writing—original draft preparation, V.P., D.T. and E.D.; writing—review and editing, V.K., G.P. and M.G.; visualization, M.G. and E.D.; supervision, V.K. All authors have read and agreed to the published version of the manuscript.

Funding: This research received no external funding.

Institutional Review Board Statement: The study was conducted in accordance with the Declaration of Helsinki and approved by the Ethics Committee of the University Hospital of Ioannina (protocol code 3263, 1 February 2019).

Informed Consent Statement: Informed consent was obtained from all subjects involved in the study.

Data Availability Statement: The data presented in this study are available upon request from the corresponding author.

Conflicts of Interest: The authors declare no conflicts of interest.

References

1. Freudenberger, H.J. Staff Burn-Out. *J. Soc. Issues* **1974**, *30*, 159–165. [CrossRef]
2. Maslach, C.; Jackson, S.E. The measurement of experienced burnout. *J. Organ. Behav.* **1981**, *2*, 99–113. [CrossRef]
3. Maslach, C.; Leiter, M.P. Understanding the burnout experience: Recent research and its implications for psychiatry. *World Psychiatry* **2016**, *15*, 103–111. [CrossRef]
4. Maslach, C.; Jackson, S.E.; Leiter, M.P. Maslach Burnout Inventory. In *Evaluating Stress: A Book of Resources*, 3rd ed.; Scarecrow Education: Lanham, MD, USA, 1997; pp. 191–218.
5. Grossi, G.; Perski, A.; Osika, W.; Savic, I. Stress-related exhaustion disorder--clinical manifestation of burnout? A review of assessment methods, sleep impairments, cognitive disturbances, and neuro-biological and physiological changes in clinical burnout. *Scand. J. Psychol.* **2015**, *56*, 626–636. [CrossRef]
6. Kelly, L.A.; Gee, P.M.; Butler, R.J. Impact of nurse burnout on organizational and position turnover. *Nurs. Outlook* **2021**, *69*, 96–102. [CrossRef]
7. Khatatbeh, H.; Pakai, A.; Al-Dwaikat, T.; Onchonga, D.; Amer, F.; Prémusz, V.; Oláh, A. Nurses' burnout and quality of life: A systematic review and critical analysis of measures used. *Nurs. Open* **2022**, *9*, 1564–1574. [CrossRef] [PubMed]
8. Bragard, I.; Dupuis, G.; Fleet, R. Quality of work life, burnout, and stress in emergency department physicians: A qualitative review. *Eur. J. Emerg. Med.* **2015**, *22*, 227–234. [CrossRef] [PubMed]
9. Sanfilippo, F.; Palumbo, G.J.; Noto, A.; Pennisi, S.; Mineri, M.; Vasile, F.; Dezio, V.; Busalacchi, D.; Murabito, P.; Astuto, M. Prevalence of burnout among intensive care physicians: A systematic review. *Rev. Bras. Ter. Intensiv.* **2020**, *32*, 458–467. [CrossRef] [PubMed]
10. Shanafelt, T.D.; Hasan, O.; Dyrbye, L.N.; Sinsky, C.; Satele, D.; Sloan, J.; West, C.P. Changes in Burnout and Satisfaction With Work-Life Balance in Physicians and the General US Working Population Between 2011 and 2014. *Mayo Clin. Proc.* **2015**, *90*, 1600–1613. [CrossRef]
11. O'Connor, K.; Muller Neff, D.; Pitman, S. Burnout in mental health professionals: A systematic review and meta-analysis of prevalence and determinants. *Eur. Psychiatry* **2018**, *53*, 74–99. [CrossRef] [PubMed]

12. Jørgensen, R.; Christensen, A.E.; Pristed, S.G.; Jepsen, I.; Telléus, G.K. Burnout in Mental Health Care Professionals Working with Inpatients in Open or Closed Wards in Psychiatric Hospitals. *Issues Ment. Health Nurs.* **2021**, *42*, 1030–1037. [CrossRef]
13. Chuang, C.H.; Tseng, P.C.; Lin, C.Y.; Lin, K.H.; Chen, Y.Y. Burnout in the intensive care unit professionals: A systematic review. *Medicine* **2016**, *95*, e5629. [CrossRef]
14. Fahrenkopf, A.M.; Sectish, T.C.; Barger, L.K.; Sharek, P.J.; Lewin, D.; Chiang, V.W.; Edwards, S.; Wiedermann, B.L.; Landrigan, C.P. Rates of medication errors among depressed and burnt out residents: Prospective cohort study. *BMJ* **2008**, *336*, 488–491. [CrossRef]
15. Tawfik, D.S.; Profit, J.; Morgenthaler, T.I.; Satele, D.V.; Sinsky, C.A.; Dyrbye, L.N.; Tutty, M.A.; West, C.P.; Shanafelt, T.D. Physician Burnout, Well-being, and Work Unit Safety Grades in Relationship to Reported Medical Errors. *Mayo Clin. Proc.* **2018**, *93*, 1571–1580. [CrossRef]
16. Dewa, C.S.; Loong, D.; Bonato, S.; Thanh, N.X.; Jacobs, P. How does burnout affect physician productivity? A systematic literature review. *BMC Health Serv. Res.* **2014**, *14*, 325. [CrossRef] [PubMed]
17. Dyrbye, L.N.; Massie, F.S., Jr.; Eacker, A.; Harper, W.; Power, D.; Durning, S.J.; Thomas, M.R.; Moutier, C.; Satele, D.; Sloan, J.; et al. Relationship between burnout and professional conduct and attitudes among US medical students. *JAMA* **2010**, *304*, 1173–1180. [CrossRef] [PubMed]
18. Rathert, C.; Williams, E.S.; Linhart, H. Evidence for the Quadruple Aim: A Systematic Review of the Literature on Physician Burnout and Patient Outcomes. *Med. Care* **2018**, *56*, 976–984. [CrossRef] [PubMed]
19. Devi, S. Doctors in distress. *Lancet* **2011**, *377*, 454–455. [CrossRef] [PubMed]
20. Williams, E.S.; Skinner, A.C. Outcomes of physician job satisfaction: A narrative review, implications, and directions for future research. *Health Care Manag. Rev.* **2003**, *28*, 119–139. [CrossRef] [PubMed]
21. Dall'Ora, C.; Ball, J.; Reinius, M.; Griffiths, P. Burnout in nursing: A theoretical review. *Hum. Resour. Health* **2020**, *18*, 41. [CrossRef] [PubMed]
22. Flannery, R.B., Jr.; Farley, E.; Tierney, T.; Walker, A.P. Characteristics of assaultive psychiatric patients: 20-year analysis of the Assaultive Staff Action Program (ASAP). *Psychiatr. Q.* **2011**, *82*, 1–10. [CrossRef]
23. Mento, C.; Silvestri, M.C.; Bruno, A.; Muscatello, M.R.A.; Cedro, C.; Pandolfo, G.; Zoccali, R.A. Workplace violence against healthcare professionals: A systematic review. *Aggress. Violent Behav.* **2020**, *51*, 101381. [CrossRef]
24. Mele, F.; Buongiorno, L.; Montalbò, D.; Ferorelli, D.; Solarino, B.; Zotti, F.; Carabellese, F.F.; Catanesi, R.; Bertolino, A.; Dell'Erba, A.; et al. Reporting Incidents in the Psychiatric Intensive Care Unit: A Retrospective Study in an Italian University Hospital. *J. Nerv. Ment. Dis.* **2022**, *210*, 622–628. [CrossRef]
25. Woo, T.; Ho, R.; Tang, A.; Tam, W. Global prevalence of burnout symptoms among nurses: A systematic review and meta-analysis. *J. Psychiatr. Res.* **2020**, *123*, 9–20. [CrossRef] [PubMed]
26. Kimo Takayesu, J.; Ramoska, E.A.; Clark, T.R.; Hansoti, B.; Dougherty, J.; Freeman, W.; Weaver, K.R.; Chang, Y.; Gross, E. Factors associated with burnout during emergency medicine residency. *Acad. Emerg. Med.* **2014**, *21*, 1031–1035. [CrossRef]
27. Rotenstein, L.S.; Torre, M.; Ramos, M.A.; Rosales, R.C.; Guille, C.; Sen, S.; Mata, D.A. Prevalence of Burnout Among Physicians: A Systematic Review. *JAMA* **2018**, *320*, 1131–1150. [CrossRef] [PubMed]
28. Dulko, D.; Zangaro, G.A. Comparison of Factors Associated with Physician and Nurse Burnout. *Nurs. Clin. N. Am.* **2022**, *57*, 53–66. [CrossRef]
29. Ntantana, A.; Matamis, D.; Savvidou, S.; Marmanidou, K.; Giannakou, M.; Gouva, M.; Nakos, G.; Koulouras, V. The impact of healthcare professionals' personality and religious beliefs on the decisions to forego life sustaining treatments: An observational, multicentre, cross-sectional study in Greek intensive care units. *BMJ Open* **2017**, *7*, e013916. [CrossRef]
30. Sikioti, T.; Zartaloudi, A.; Pappa, D.; Mangoulia, P.; Fradelos, E.C.; Kourti, F.E.; Koutelekos, I.; Dousis, E.; Margari, N.; Stavropoulou, A.; et al. Stress and burnout among Greek critical care nurses during the COVID-19 pandemic. *AIMS Public Health* **2023**, *10*, 755–774. [CrossRef] [PubMed]
31. van Mol, M.M.; Kompanje, E.J.; Benoit, D.D.; Bakker, J.; Nijkamp, M.D. The Prevalence of Compassion Fatigue and Burnout among Healthcare Professionals in Intensive Care Units: A Systematic Review. *PLoS ONE* **2015**, *10*, e0136955. [CrossRef]
32. McManus, I.C.; Keeling, A.; Paice, E. Stress, burnout and doctors' attitudes to work are determined by personality and learning style: A twelve year longitudinal study of UK medical graduates. *BMC Med.* **2004**, *2*, 29. [CrossRef]
33. Eysenck, H. *Personality Psychology in Europe: Theoretical and Empirical Developments*; Bonarius, H., Van Heck, G., Smid, N., Eds.; Swets & Zeitlinger: Lisse, The Netherlands, 1984.
34. Maher, B.A.; Maher, W.B. Personality and psychopathology: A historical perspective. *J. Abnorm. Psychol.* **1994**, *103*, 72–77. [CrossRef]
35. Eysenck, H.J.; Eysenck, S.B.G. *Manual of the Eysenck Personality Questionnaire: (EPQ-R Adult)*; EdITS/Educational and Industrial Testing Service San Diego, Calif.: San Diego, CA, USA, 1994.
36. Eysenck, H.J.; Eysenck, M.W. *Personality and Individual Differences: A Natural Science Approach*; Eysenck, H.J., Eysenck, M.W., Eds.; Plenum Press: New York, NY, USA, 1985.
37. Eysenck, H.J.; Eysenck, S.B.G. The Orthogonality of Psychoticism and Neuroticism: A Factorial Study. *Percept. Mot. Ski.* **1971**, *33*, 461–462. [CrossRef]
38. Angelini, G. Big five model personality traits and job burnout: A systematic literature review. *BMC Psychol.* **2023**, *11*, 49. [CrossRef] [PubMed]

39. Brown, P.A.; Slater, M.; Lofters, A. Personality and burnout among primary care physicians: An international study. *Psychol. Res. Behav. Manag.* **2019**, *12*, 169–177. [CrossRef] [PubMed]
40. Divinakumar, K.J.; Bhat, P.S.; Prakash, J.; Srivastava, K. Personality traits and its correlation to burnout in female nurses. *Ind. Psychiatry J.* **2019**, *28*, 24–28. [CrossRef] [PubMed]
41. Grigorescu, S.; Cazan, A.M.; Grigorescu, O.D.; Rogozea, L.M. The role of the personality traits and work characteristics in the prediction of the burnout syndrome among nurses—A new approach within predictive, preventive, and personalized medicine concept. *EPMA J.* **2018**, *9*, 355–365. [CrossRef]
42. Narang, G.; Wymer, K.; Mi, L.; Wolter, C.; Humphreys, M.; Stern, K. Personality Traits and Burnout: A Survey of Practicing US Urologists. *Urology* **2022**, *167*, 43–48. [CrossRef] [PubMed]
43. Prins, D.J.; van Vendeloo, S.N.; Brand, P.L.P.; Van der Velpen, I.; de Jong, K.; van den Heijkant, F.; Van der Heijden, F.; Prins, J.T. The relationship between burnout, personality traits, and medical specialty. A national study among Dutch residents. *Med. Teach.* **2019**, *41*, 584–590. [CrossRef]
44. Louwen, C.; Reidlinger, D.; Milne, N. Profiling health professionals' personality traits, behaviour styles and emotional intelligence: A systematic review. *BMC Med. Educ.* **2023**, *23*, 120. [CrossRef]
45. Atherton, O.E.; Willroth, E.C.; Graham, E.K.; Luo, J.; Mroczek, D.K.; Lewis-Thames, M.W. Rural-urban differences in personality traits and well-being in adulthood. *J. Pers.* **2024**, *92*, 73–87. [CrossRef]
46. Weidmann, R.; Chopik, W.J. Explicating narrow and broad conceptualizations of environmental influences on personality. *J. Pers.* **2024**, *92*, 5–15. [CrossRef]
47. Probst, J.C.; Laditka, S.B.; Moore, C.G.; Harun, N.; Powell, M.P.; Baxley, E.G. Rural-urban differences in depression prevalence: Implications for family medicine. *Fam. Med.* **2006**, *38*, 653–660.
48. van den Bosch, M.; Meyer-Lindenberg, A. Environmental Exposures and Depression: Biological Mechanisms and Epidemiological Evidence. *Annu. Rev. Public Health* **2019**, *40*, 239–259. [CrossRef]
49. van Os, J.; Kenis, G.; Rutten, B.P. The environment and schizophrenia. *Nature* **2010**, *468*, 203–212. [CrossRef]
50. Szyszkowicz, M.; Rowe, B.H.; Colman, I. Air pollution and daily emergency department visits for depression. *Int. J. Occup. Med. Environ. Health* **2009**, *22*, 355–362. [CrossRef]
51. Power, M.C.; Kioumourtzoglou, M.A.; Hart, J.E.; Okereke, O.I.; Laden, F.; Weisskopf, M.G. The relation between past exposure to fine particulate air pollution and prevalent anxiety: Observational cohort study. *BMJ* **2015**, *350*, h1111. [CrossRef] [PubMed]
52. Newbury, J.B.; Arseneault, L.; Beevers, S.; Kitwiroon, N.; Roberts, S.; Pariante, C.M.; Kelly, F.J.; Fisher, H.L. Association of Air Pollution Exposure With Psychotic Experiences During Adolescence. *JAMA Psychiatry* **2019**, *76*, 614–623. [CrossRef] [PubMed]
53. EEA-JRC. *Environment and Human Health: Joint EEA-JRC Report*; EUR-OP: Luxembourg, 2013.
54. iMEdDLAB. Beds and Nursing Staff per COVID ICU. 2021. Available online: https://lab.imedd.org/ypostelexosi-meth-covid-thnitotita-plirotita-esy (accessed on 14 January 2024).
55. Anagnostopoulos, F.; Papadatou, D. Factorial composition and internal consistency of the Greek version of the Maslach Burnout Inventory. *Psychol. Them.* **1992**, *5*, 183–202.
56. Dimitriou, E. EPQ personality questionnaire. Greek validation in the Greek population. *Engefalos* **1986**, *23*, 41–54.
57. Donias, S.; Karastergiou, A.; Manos, N. Standardization of the symptom checklist-90-R rating scale in a Greek population. *Psychiatriki* **1991**, *2*, 42–48.
58. Zis, P.; Anagnostopoulos, F.; Sykioti, P. Burnout in medical residents: A study based on the job demands-resources model. *Sci. World J.* **2014**, *2014*, 673279. [CrossRef]
59. Derogatis, L.R. *SCL 90 R Administration, Scoring and Procedures Manual II for the Revised Version and Other Instruments of the Psychopathology Rating Scale Series*; Clinical Psychometric Research: Towson, MD, USA, 1986.
60. Cronbach, L.J.; Meehl, P.E. Construct validity in psychological tests. *Psychol. Bull.* **1955**, *52*, 281–302. [CrossRef]
61. Hayes, A.F. *Introduction to Mediation, Moderation, and Conditional Process Analysis: A Regression-Based Approach (Methodology in the Social Sciences)*, 2nd ed.; The Guilford Press New York: New York, NY, USA, 2018.
62. R Core Team. *R: A Language and Environment for Statistical Computing*; R Foundation for Statistical Computing: Vienna, Austria, 2021; Available online: www.R-project.org (accessed on 14 January 2024).
63. Aluja, A.; García, Ó.; García, L.F. A psychometric analysis of the revised Eysenck Personality Questionnaire short scale. *Personal. Individ. Differ.* **2003**, *35*, 449–460. [CrossRef]
64. Lewis, C.A.; Francis, L.J.; Shevlin, M.; Forrest, S. Confirmatory factor analysis of the French translation of the abbreviated form of the revised Eysenck Personality Questionnaire (EPQR-A). *Eur. J. Psychol. Assess.* **2002**, *18*, 179–185. [CrossRef]
65. Escorial, S.; Navas, M.J. Analysis of the Gender Variable in the Eysenck Personality Questionnaire–Revised Scales Using Differential Item Functioning Techniques. *Educ. Psychol. Meas.* **2007**, *67*, 990–1001. [CrossRef]
66. Forrest, S.; Lewis, C.A.; Shevlin, M. Examining the factor structure and differential functioning of the Eysenck personality questionnaire revised–abbreviated. *Personal. Individ. Differ.* **2000**, *29*, 579–588. [CrossRef]
67. Costa, P.T.; McCrae, R.R. Four ways five factors are basic. *Personal. Individ. Differ.* **1992**, *13*, 653–665. [CrossRef]
68. Kennedy, B.; Curtis, K.; Waters, D. Is there a relationship between personality and choice of nursing specialty: An integrative literature review. *BMC Nurs.* **2014**, *13*, 40. [CrossRef] [PubMed]
69. Levine, C.D.; Wilson, S.F.; Guido, G.W. Personality factors of critical care nurses. *Heart Lung* **1988**, *17*, 392–398. [PubMed]

70. Scheepers, F.E.; de Mul, J.; Boer, F.; Hoogendijk, W.J. Psychosis as an Evolutionary Adaptive Mechanism to Changing Environments. *Front. Psychiatry* **2018**, *9*, 237. [CrossRef]
71. Nyhagen, R.; Egerod, I.; Rustøen, T.; Lerdal, A.; Kirkevold, M. Unidentified communication challenges in the intensive care unit: A qualitative study using multiple triangulations. *Aust. Crit. Care* **2023**, *36*, 215–222. [CrossRef]
72. Ten Hoorn, S.; Elbers, P.W.; Girbes, A.R.; Tuinman, P.R. Communicating with conscious and mechanically ventilated critically ill patients: A systematic review. *Crit. Care* **2016**, *20*, 333. [CrossRef] [PubMed]
73. Baumgarten, M.; Poulsen, I. Patients' experiences of being mechanically ventilated in an ICU: A qualitative metasynthesis. *Scand. J. Caring Sci.* **2015**, *29*, 205–214. [CrossRef] [PubMed]
74. Karlsson, V.; Lindahl, B.; Bergbom, I. Patients' statements and experiences concerning receiving mechanical ventilation: A prospective video-recorded study. *Nurs. Inq.* **2012**, *19*, 247–258. [CrossRef]
75. Ayuso-Murillo, D.; Colomer-Sánchez, A.; Herrera-Peco, I. Communication skills in ICU and adult hospitalisation unit nursing staff. *Enferm. Intensiv.* **2017**, *28*, 105–113. [CrossRef] [PubMed]
76. Adams, A.; Mannix, T.; Harrington, A. Nurses' communication with families in the intensive care unit–a literature review. *Nurs. Crit. Care* **2017**, *22*, 70–80. [CrossRef]
77. Ormel, J.; Jeronimus, B.F.; Kotov, R.; Riese, H.; Bos, E.H.; Hankin, B.; Rosmalen, J.G.M.; Oldehinkel, A.J. Neuroticism and common mental disorders: Meaning and utility of a complex relationship. *Clin. Psychol. Rev.* **2013**, *33*, 686–697. [CrossRef] [PubMed]
78. Li, W.W.; Xie, G. Personality and job satisfaction among Chinese health practitioners: The mediating role of professional quality of life. *Health Psychol. Open* **2020**, *7*, 2055102920965053. [CrossRef] [PubMed]
79. Lu, M.; Zhang, F.; Tang, X.; Wang, L.; Zan, J.; Zhu, Y.; Feng, D. Do type A personality and neuroticism moderate the relationships of occupational stressors, job satisfaction and burnout among Chinese older nurses? A cross-sectional survey. *BMC Nurs.* **2022**, *21*, 88. [CrossRef]
80. Myhren, H.; Ekeberg, O.; Stokland, O. Job Satisfaction and Burnout among Intensive Care Unit Nurses and Physicians. *Crit. Care Res. Pract.* **2013**, *2013*, 786176. [CrossRef] [PubMed]
81. Papazian, L.; Hraiech, S.; Loundou, A.; Herridge, M.S.; Boyer, L. High-level burnout in physicians and nurses working in adult ICUs: A systematic review and meta-analysis. *Intensive Care Med.* **2023**, *49*, 387–400. [CrossRef] [PubMed]
82. Ramírez-Elvira, S.; Romero-Béjar, J.L.; Suleiman-Martos, N.; Gómez-Urquiza, J.L.; Monsalve-Reyes, C.; Cañadas-De la Fuente, G.A.; Albendín-García, L. Prevalence, Risk Factors and Burnout Levels in Intensive Care Unit Nurses: A Systematic Review and Meta-Analysis. *Int. J. Environ. Res. Public Health* **2021**, *18*, 11432. [CrossRef] [PubMed]
83. Leiter, M.P.; Spence Laschinger, H.K. Relationships of work and practice environment to professional burnout: Testing a causal model. *Nurs. Res.* **2006**, *55*, 137–146. [CrossRef]
84. Asl, R.G.; Taghinejad, R.; Parizad, N.; Jasemi, M. The Relationship Between Professional Autonomy and Job Stress Among Intensive Care Unit Nurses: A Descriptive Correlational Study. *Iran. J. Nurs. Midwifery Res.* **2022**, *27*, 119–124. [CrossRef] [PubMed]
85. Bégat, I.; Ellefsen, B.; Severinsson, E. Nurses' satisfaction with their work environment and the outcomes of clinical nursing supervision on nurses' experiences of well-being—A Norwegian study. *J. Nurs. Manag.* **2005**, *13*, 221–230. [CrossRef]
86. Krukowska-Sitek, H.; Krupa, S.; Grad, I. The Impact of the COVID-19 Pandemic on the Professional Autonomy of Anesthesiological Nurses and Trust in the Therapeutic Team of Intensive Therapy Units-Polish Multicentre Study. *Int. J. Environ. Res. Public Health* **2022**, *19*, 12755. [CrossRef] [PubMed]
87. Carrillo-García, C.; Solano-Ruíz Mdel, C.; Martínez-Roche, M.E.; Gómez-García, C.I. Job satisfaction among health care workers: The role of gender and age. *Rev. Lat. Am. Enferm.* **2013**, *21*, 1314–1320. [CrossRef]
88. Padilla Fortunatti, C.; Palmeiro-Silva, Y.K. Effort-Reward Imbalance and Burnout Among ICU Nursing Staff: A Cross-Sectional Study. *Nurs. Res.* **2017**, *66*, 410–416. [CrossRef]
89. Poncet, M.C.; Toullic, P.; Papazian, L.; Kentish-Barnes, N.; Timsit, J.F.; Pochard, F.; Chevret, S.; Schlemmer, B.; Azoulay, E. Burnout syndrome in critical care nursing staff. *Am. J. Respir. Crit. Care Med.* **2007**, *175*, 698–704. [CrossRef]
90. Kashtanov, A.; Molotok, E.; Yavorovskiy, A.; Boyarkov, A.; Vasil'ev, Y.; Alsaegh, A.; Dydykin, S.; Kytko, O.; Meylanova, R.; Enina, Y.; et al. A Comparative Cross-Sectional Study Assessing the Psycho-Emotional State of Intensive Care Units' Physicians and Nurses of COVID-19 Hospitals of a Russian Metropolis. *Int. J. Environ. Res. Public Health* **2022**, *19*, 1828. [CrossRef] [PubMed]
91. Hall, C.E.; Milward, J.; Spoiala, C.; Bhogal, J.K.; Weston, D.; Potts, H.W.W.; Caulfield, T.; Toolan, M.; Kanga, K.; El-Sheikha, S.; et al. The mental health of staff working on intensive care units over the COVID-19 winter surge of 2020 in England: A cross sectional survey. *Br. J. Anaesth.* **2022**, *128*, 971–979. [CrossRef] [PubMed]
92. Dragioti, E.; Tsartsalis, D.; Mentis, M.; Mantzoukas, S.; Gouva, M. Impact of the COVID-19 pandemic on the mental health of hospital staff: An umbrella review of 44 meta-analyses. *Int. J. Nurs. Stud.* **2022**, *131*, 104272. [CrossRef] [PubMed]
93. Aslanidis, V.; Tsolaki, V.; Papadonta, M.E.; Amanatidis, T.; Parisi, K.; Makris, D.; Zakynthinos, E. The Impact of the COVID-19 Pandemic on Mental Health and Quality of Life in COVID-19 Department Healthcare Workers in Central Greece. *J. Pers. Med.* **2023**, *13*, 250. [CrossRef]
94. Blekas, A.; Voitsidis, P.; Athanasiadou, M.; Parlapani, E.; Chatzigeorgiou, A.F.; Skoupra, M.; Syngelakis, M.; Holeva, V.; Diakogiannis, I. COVID-19: PTSD symptoms in Greek health care professionals. *Psychol. Trauma.* **2020**, *12*, 812–819. [CrossRef] [PubMed]

95. Mavrovounis, G.; Mavrovouni, D.; Mermiri, M.; Papadaki, P.; Chalkias, A.; Zarogiannis, S.; Christodoulou, N.; Gourgoulianis, K.; Pantazopoulos, I. Watch Out for Burnout in COVID-19: A Greek Health Care Personnel Study. *Inquiry* **2022**, *59*, 469580221097829. [CrossRef]
96. Milas, G.P.; Issaris, V.; Zareifopoulos, N. Burnout for medical professionals during the COVID-19 pandemic in Greece; the role of primary care. *Hosp Pr.* **2022**, *50*, 102–103. [CrossRef] [PubMed]
97. Benincasa, V.; Passannante, M.; Perrini, F.; Carpinelli, L.; Moccia, G.; Marinaci, T.; Capunzo, M.; Pironti, C.; Genovese, A.; Savarese, G.; et al. Burnout and Psychological Vulnerability in First Responders: Monitoring Depersonalization and Phobic Anxiety during the COVID-19 Pandemic. *Int. J. Environ. Res. Public Health* **2022**, *19*, 2794. [CrossRef]
98. Hou, J.; Xu, B.; Zhang, J.; Luo, L.; Pen, X.; Chen, S.; Ma, G.; Hu, Z.; Kong, X. Psychological Status and Job Burnout of Nurses Working in the Frontline of the Novel Coronavirus in China During the Delta Variant Outbreak: A Cross-Sectional Survey. *Psychol. Res. Behav. Manag.* **2022**, *15*, 533–546. [CrossRef]
99. Rössler, W.; Hengartner, M.P.; Ajdacic-Gross, V.; Angst, J. Predictors of burnout: Results from a prospective community study. *Eur. Arch. Psychiatry Clin. Neurosci.* **2015**, *265*, 19–25. [CrossRef]
100. Saulsman, L.M.; Page, A.C. The five-factor model and personality disorder empirical literature: A meta-analytic review. *Clin. Psychol. Rev.* **2004**, *23*, 1055–1085. [CrossRef] [PubMed]
101. Strickhouser, J.E.; Zell, E.; Krizan, Z. Does personality predict health and well-being? A metasynthesis. *Health Psychol.* **2017**, *36*, 797–810. [CrossRef] [PubMed]
102. Lederbogen, F.; Kirsch, P.; Haddad, L.; Streit, F.; Tost, H.; Schuch, P.; Wüst, S.; Pruessner, J.C.; Rietschel, M.; Deuschle, M.; et al. City living and urban upbringing affect neural social stress processing in humans. *Nature* **2011**, *474*, 498–501. [CrossRef] [PubMed]
103. Peen, J.; Schoevers, R.A.; Beekman, A.T.; Dekker, J. The current status of urban-rural differences in psychiatric disorders. *Acta Psychiatr. Scand.* **2010**, *121*, 84–93. [CrossRef] [PubMed]
104. Shanafelt, T.D.; Boone, S.; Tan, L.; Dyrbye, L.N.; Sotile, W.; Satele, D.; West, C.P.; Sloan, J.; Oreskovich, M.R. Burnout and satisfaction with work-life balance among US physicians relative to the general US population. *Arch. Intern. Med.* **2012**, *172*, 1377–1385. [CrossRef]
105. West, C.P.; Dyrbye, L.N.; Erwin, P.J.; Shanafelt, T.D. Interventions to prevent and reduce physician burnout: A systematic review and meta-analysis. *Lancet* **2016**, *388*, 2272–2281. [CrossRef]
106. West, C.P.; Dyrbye, L.N.; Sinsky, C.; Trockel, M.; Tutty, M.; Nedelec, L.; Carlasare, L.E.; Shanafelt, T.D. Resilience and Burnout Among Physicians and the General US Working Population. *JAMA Netw. Open* **2020**, *3*, e209385. [CrossRef]
107. West, C.P.; Shanafelt, T.D.; Kolars, J.C. Quality of life, burnout, educational debt, and medical knowledge among internal medicine residents. *JAMA* **2011**, *306*, 952–960. [CrossRef]
108. Xing, J.; Sun, N.; Xu, J.; Geng, S.; Li, Y. Study of the mental health status of medical personnel dealing with new coronavirus pneumonia. *PLoS ONE* **2020**, *15*, e0233145. [CrossRef]
109. Pachi, A.; Kavourgia, E.; Bratis, D.; Fytsilis, K.; Papageorgiou, S.M.; Lekka, D.; Sikaras, C.; Tselebis, A. Anger and Aggression in Relation to Psychological Resilience and Alcohol Abuse among Health Professionals during the First Pandemic Wave. *Healthcare* **2023**, *11*, 2031. [CrossRef]
110. Flannery, L.; Ramjan, L.M.; Peters, K. End-of-life decisions in the Intensive Care Unit (ICU)—Exploring the experiences of ICU nurses and doctors—A critical literature review. *Aust. Crit. Care* **2016**, *29*, 97–103. [CrossRef] [PubMed]
111. Van den Bulcke, B.; Metaxa, V.; Reyners, A.K.; Rusinova, K.; Jensen, H.I.; Malmgren, J.; Darmon, M.; Talmor, D.; Meert, A.P.; Cancelliere, L.; et al. Ethical climate and intention to leave among critical care clinicians: An observational study in 68 intensive care units across Europe and the United States. *Intensive Care Med.* **2020**, *46*, 46–56. [CrossRef]
112. Moss, M.; Good, V.S.; Gozal, D.; Kleinpell, R.; Sessler, C.N. An Official Critical Care Societies Collaborative Statement-Burnout Syndrome in Critical Care Health-care Professionals: A Call for Action. *Chest* **2016**, *150*, 17–26. [CrossRef] [PubMed]
113. De Hert, S. Burnout in Healthcare Workers: Prevalence, Impact and Preventative Strategies. *Local. Reg. Anesth.* **2020**, *13*, 171–183. [CrossRef] [PubMed]
114. Garcia, C.L.; Abreu, L.C.; Ramos, J.L.S.; Castro, C.F.D.; Smiderle, F.R.N.; Santos, J.A.D.; Bezerra, I.M.P. Influence of Burnout on Patient Safety: Systematic Review and Meta-Analysis. *Medicina* **2019**, *55*, 553. [CrossRef]
115. Ryu, I.S.; Shim, J. The Influence of Burnout on Patient Safety Management Activities of Shift Nurses: The Mediating Effect of Compassion Satisfaction. *Int. J. Environ. Res. Public Health* **2021**, *18*, 12210. [CrossRef]
116. Welp, A.; Meier, L.L.; Manser, T. Emotional exhaustion and workload predict clinician-rated and objective patient safety. *Front. Psychol.* **2014**, *5*, 1573. [CrossRef]
117. Haas, J.S.; Cook, E.F.; Puopolo, A.L.; Burstin, H.R.; Cleary, P.D.; Brennan, T.A. Is the professional satisfaction of general internists associated with patient satisfaction? *J. Gen. Intern. Med.* **2000**, *15*, 122–128. [CrossRef]

Disclaimer/Publisher's Note: The statements, opinions and data contained in all publications are solely those of the individual author(s) and contributor(s) and not of MDPI and/or the editor(s). MDPI and/or the editor(s) disclaim responsibility for any injury to people or property resulting from any ideas, methods, instructions or products referred to in the content.

Case Report

A Fatal Case of Presumptive Diagnosis of Leptospirosis Involving the Central Nervous System

Christina Alexopoulou [1,*], Athanasia Proklou [1], Sofia Kokkini [1], Maria Raissaki [2], Ioannis Konstantinou [1] and Eumorfia Kondili [1]

1. Department of Intensive Care Medicine, University Hospital of Heraklion, 71500 Heraklion, Greece; proklath@gmail.com (A.P.); sofkok@hotmail.com (S.K.); konstantinou.ioannis@yahoo.gr (I.K.); kondylie@uoc.gr (E.K.)
2. Radiology Department, University Hospital of Heraklion, 71500 Heraklion, Greece; mraissaki@yahoo.gr
* Correspondence: calexopoulou@pagni.gr; Tel.: +30-281-039-2414

Abstract: Leptospirosis is a reemerging zooanthroponosis with a worldwide distribution, though it has a higher incidence in areas with tropical climate. A characteristic finding of the disease is its wide spectrum of symptoms and organ involvement, as it can appear either with very mild flu-like manifestations or with multiorgan failure, affecting the central nervous system (CNS) with a concomitant hepatorenal dysfunction (Weil's syndrome) and significant high mortality rate. We report herein a fatal case of a 25 years old female, previously healthy, with impaired neurological status. She had high fever and severe multiorgan failure. The clinical data and the epidemiological factors were not conclusive for the diagnosis, and the first serology test from the cerebrospinal fluid (CSF) and sera samples were negative. When the repetition of the blood test showed elevated IgM antibodies, Leptospirosis was the presumptive diagnosis. Although CNS involvement is rare, the diagnosis should be considered when there is an elevated risk of exposure. The diagnostic protocol should encompass direct evidence of the bacterium and indirect measurement of antibodies. Timely detection and management are imperative to forestall complications and fatality associated with the disease.

Keywords: Leptospirosis; CNS; coma; Weil's syndrome; case report

1. Introduction

Leptospirosis is a reemerging zooanthroponosis caused by spirochetes of the genus *Leptospira*. Different ancient reports from the Far East had described febrile icteric illness, probably leptospirosis, as a 'rice field jaundice' in the rice-harvesting Chinese population, or as 'Akiyami (autumn fever)' in Japan. Moreover, in European texts, the disease was described as 'cane-cutter's disease' or 'swineherd's disease' [1]. In 1886, Adolph Weil in Heidelberg described leptospirosis as a syndrome with multiorgan manifestations, high fever, concomitant icterus, enlarged spleen, acute renal impairment, and conjunctivitis. The causative organism was demonstrated a few years later by Stimson, who identified it by silver staining the presence of clumps of spirochetes in the kidney tubules of a patient who died of yellow fever. Stimson named them *Spirochaeta interrogans*, from their hooked ends resembling a question mark [1,2].

Though the distribution of leptospirosis is worldwide, an incidence rate of more than 10 cases per 100,000 of the population is recorded in tropical climates and significantly less (0.1–1 per 100,000) in temperate climates [3]. East Sub-Saharan Africa, the Caribbean, Oceania, and South East Asia are related, with more than 70% of reported cases of leptospirosis. While the worldwide prevalence of the disease has remained stable, it tends to occur more frequently following natural disasters such as flooding or earthquakes. Extended periods of hot, dry weather can also lead to increased leptospires in freshwater ponds and rivers, making swimming, canoeing, white water rafting, fishing, and other water sports potential risk factors for outbreaks. Young individuals who work in farming and are in contact with livestock and those exposed to rodents at their workplaces, particularly males, are at a higher risk of infection [4].

Although any mammal can be an animal reservoir for the organism, small mammals are the most important maintenance hosts, as they can transfer the pathogen to domestic farm animals, dogs, and humans through urine. The transmission of leptospirosis to humans occurs by direct exposure to the urine of infected animals or urine-contaminated water and soil. This can happen through recreational or occupational activities. The contaminated water or soil infects humans via abrasions or cuts in the skin, the conjunctiva, or the gastrointestinal route. Prolonged water immersion can also lead to infection, particularly if skin abrasion occurs. In rare instances, transmission can also occur through inhalation of infected water or aerosols through the mucous membranes of the respiratory tract or following an animal bite [2]. Although human-to-human transmission is uncommon, there have been reports of transmission during sexual intercourse [5].

Leptospirosis is frequently underdiagnosed as it can manifest through a broad spectrum of nonspecific signs and symptoms that involve multiple organs. In certain geographic locations, a mild, self-limiting, acute febrile illness may be present, while in tropical and high-risk areas, a severe, life-threatening form with multiple organ failure is described. Dengue and other hemorrhagic fevers, rickettsial infection, malaria, and even common bacterial sepsis, can be confused with the initial presentation of leptospirosis. The most common presentation of the infection is the anicteric form, resembling seasonal influenza, while icterohemorrhagic leptospirosis, or Weil's syndrome, represents the most severe form of the disease with significant morbidity and mortality of 40%. About 10% of the infected population will develop a severe form of the disease [6].

The incubation period can vary from 2–20 days, with a mean range between 7–12 days. The disease often has a biphasic clinical presentation with an acute or leptospiremic phase occurring in the first week, followed by an 'immune phase' [7]. During the first phase, fever, myalgias (especially in the paraspinal muscles with signs of meningism, or the abdominal muscles), chills, and headache (with retro-orbital pain and photophobia) are the main nonspecific symptoms. On the third to fourth day, conjunctival suffusion, and less often a transient skin rash, can be presented. The second phase of the disease is characterized by IgM production, blood release, and excretion of leptospires in the urine, as spirochaetes settle in the proximal tubules of the kidney. During this phase of the disease, most complications can occur depending on the degree of organ involvement and the virulence of the organism [6]. The exact pathogenetic mechanisms of the most severe form of the disease are not completely understood yet, and the most severe form of the disease is thought as a form of vasculitis. The clinical presentation includes jaundice as a prominent feature, and severe septic shock with multiple acute organ involvement, mainly kidneys, brain, and lungs. Death is often related to multiple organ failure and diffuse alveolar hemorrhaging. Leptospirosis involves the nervous system in around 10–15% of the cases, mainly in the form of aseptic meningitis. However, other atypical forms of nervous system involvement can also occur, including intracranial bleeding and thrombosis, Guillain–Barré syndrome, and ocular manifestations in the form of uveitis and optic neuritis [8]. Diagnosis of leptospirosis is challenging in many cases. It is based on suggestive clinical symptoms with a history of risk exposure. Increased clinical suspicion is crucial for the severe form of the disease. We report herein a case of a 25-year-old female who presented with Weil's syndrome and severe brain involvement. Despite targeted therapy, the patient died from multi-organ failure.

2. Case Description

A 25-year-old female with an unremarkable past medical history was transferred to the emergency department of a regional insular hospital of Greece after an abrupt loss of consciousness and a fainting episode in a public place, unconscious with a Glasgow Coma Scale (GCS) 6/15, febrile (40 °C body temperature), and a macular degenerative hemorrhagic rash of the forehead and periocular areas. She was intubated, and a brain Computed Tomography (CT) scan was performed with unremarkable findings. A lumbar puncture was performed, and both cerebrospinal fluid (CSF) biochemical and microbiological tests were normal. Specifically, the CSF investigation included the following: cytology: 10 cells per field of view, 7680 red blood cells per field of view, microbiology: Gram stain was negative, as was the culture and biochemistry: glucose ratio (CSF/blood) was 55% (reference range for normal above 50%), and protein was 35 mg/dL (reference range 15–45 mg/dl); polymerase chain reaction (PCR) for common encephalitis-meningitis pathogens was negative and included the following: *Cytomegalovirus (CMV), Varicella Zoster virus (VZV), Herpes Simplex virus 1/2 (HSV1/2), Epstein–Barr virus (EBV), Herpex virus 6 (HHV6), Enterovirus, Parechovirus, Escherichia coli k1, Haemophilus influenzae, Listeria monocytogenes, Neisseria meningitidis, Streptococcus agalactiae, Streptococcus pneumoniae*, and *Cryptococcus neoformans/gattii*.

The patient was initially admitted to the Intensive Care Unit (ICU) of the insular regional hospital. One day later, she was transferred to the ICU of our University Hospital for advanced organ support due to clinical deterioration and multiple organ failure. During her admission, she appeared on substantial hemodynamic instability on norepinephrine 0.5 mcg/kg/min and tachycardia (120 rpm). At that time, aggressive fluid resuscitation, vasopressor, and empirical broad-spectrum antibiotic therapy (cefepime [Zefepime, Vocate] 2 gr twice per day and vancomycin [Voxin, Vianex] 2 gr continuous infusion) were started for presumed septic shock. Initial investigations revealed severe thrombocytopenia (8 K/μL, reference values 150–450 K/μL), elevated creatinine kinase enzyme (CPK = 5520 U/L, reference values < 172 U/L), elevated international normalized ratio (INR = 2.66, reference values 0.85–1.2) and D-dimers > 35.20 (reference values 0–0.55 mg/L), low fibrinogen levels (128.1, reference values 210–400 mg/dL), elevated liver function tests (alanine transaminase 362 U/L (reference values < 35 U/L), and aspartate aminotransferase 562 U/L (reference values < 35 U/L) and mild renal impairment.

On admission to our department, differential diagnosis included a wide range of diseases which had to be excluded. The main symptoms, laboratory tests, and results for the first eight days are summarized at Table 1. The patient presented acute liver and renal failure, severe thrombocytopenia, CNS involvement, and non-generalized rash consisted of non-palpable purpura localized around the left eye-periorbital and on the left breast accompanied with ecchymosis.

Laboratory results for autoimmune diseases were as follows: ANA 1:20 (negative, reference range < 1:20), ANCA 1:80 (negative, reference range < 1:80), RF <10.1 (negative, reference ratio 0–35 IU/mL), Anti B2-GPI IgM 0.36 (negative, reference range < 12 U/mL), Anti B2-GPI IgG 1.61 U/mL, reference range < 12 U/mL), C4: 15 mg/dL (reference range 15–47 mg/dL), C3: 88 mg/dL (reference range 87–187 mg/dL), IgM: 74,60 mg/dL (reference range 25–170 mg/dL), IgG: 765 mg/dL (reference range 701–1600 mg/dL), and IgA: 151 mg/dL (reference range 48–368 mg/dL). Autoimmune diseases, mainly systemic lupus erythematosus (SLE) vasculitis, were excluded based on negative laboratory results (ANA, ANCA, etc.) and on the absence of arthritis, generalized rash, and other diagnostic criteria. Purpura was attributed to the severe underlying thrombocytopenia. The urine sediment findings were consistent with acute kidney injury without any signs of glomerulonephritis or interstitial nephritis, and were attributed to the substantial hemodynamic instability on presentation and possibly during the transfer of the patient. The low complement levels (54.7 mg/dL, reference values 87–187 mg/dL), as well as the high levels of ferritin (5066 ng/mL, reference values 4.63–204 ng/mL), were attributed to acute liver failure, and were restored in the next days of hospitalization. Veno-occlusive disease was excluded by an abdomen computed tomography angiography (CTA).

A full-body CT scan revealed unremarkable findings, except for ground glass with concomitant consolidation mainly on the left lung and to a lesser extent on the right lower lobe. Abdominal organs presented normal on the CT scan without hepatomegaly or splenomegaly. All CT scans were performed on a 128-slice CT scanner (Revolution GSI; GE Healthcare, Chicago, IL, USA).

Table 1. Main symptoms, laboratory tests and results during the first 8 days.

Day 0 Hospital in rural area	Coma, fever (40 °C), meningism, and a macular degenerative hemorrhagic rash of the forehead and periocular areas Respiratory failure	Brain CT scan Lumbar puncture	Normal
		PCR of CSF for common pathogens	Negative
Day 1 Our hospital	Transfer to our hospital Severe shock Acute liver and renal failure, severe thrombocytopenia, non-palpable purpura localized around the left eye-periorbital and on the left breast accompanied with ecchymosis.	Cultures: Blood, Bronchial specimen, urine Broad serological tests Blood ImmunoDOT Leptospira test	All negative
		ANA ANCA Anti B2-GPI IgM Anti B2-GPI IgG C3, C4, IgM, IgG, IgA	All normal
Day 2	Intubated Hemodynamically stable High clinical suspicion of legionella	CT angiography of brain abdomen Lumbar puncture Bone marrow biopsy	All normal
Day 5	Analgosedation discontinuation Myoclonus Exophoria Coma	Brain MRI	Cytotoxic edema in the context of global hypoxic-ischemic injury
Day 8	No improvement	Blood ImmunoDOT Leptospira test	Elevated IgM

However, no schistocytes were revealed on peripheral blood smear. The blood, urine and bronchial specimen's cultures revealed no pathogen. The blood culture system used was BacT/ALERT, in bottle types BacT/ALERT FA PLUS and BacT/ALERT FN PLUS containing aerobic and anaerobic media, respectively, with adsorbent polymeric resin beads. The method used for monitoring growth was colorimetric change caused by a drop in pH from increased CO_2 levels. Urine cultures were inoculated in Drigalski Agar, Columbia ANC agar +5% sheep blood and Trypticase™ Soy Agar, BD Diagnostics. Bronchial specimens were inoculated in Columbia agar +5% sheep blood and Chocolate Agar with Vitox.

A broad serological testing was carried out including *CMV, Hepatitis A virus (HAV), VZV, Adenovirus, Parvovirus, Echovirus, Coxsackie, HSV1/2, Measles, Hepatitis C virus (HCV), Hepatitis B virus (HBV), Human Immunodeficiency virus (HIV), EBV Rickettsia typhi, Rickettsia conorii, Trichinella, Cryptococcus species, Brucella (Wright/Rose Bengal), Treponema (PRP), Salmonella (WIDAL), Borellia burgdorferi, Bordetella pertussis, Plasmodium, Leishmania,* and *Leptospira.* All results were negative.

Based on hematologist consultation, a bone marrow biopsy was performed to exclude acute hemophagocytic syndrome. The peripheral blood smear revealed 88% neutrophils, 5% lypmphocytes, and 6% monocytes with a total number of 6.400 K/μL WBCs. Schistocytes, two per field of view and two erythroblasts per field of view were also present. Phagocytosis in bone marrow was present in the bone marrow smear. The bone marrow biopsy showed hematopoietic marrow normal, in relation to age and cellularity (the hematopoietic cellular elements accounted for about 50–55% of the area of myelochores). All three hematopoietic lines were recognized with a ratio of medullary to rubella 2/1. Normal maturation of medullary. Normal number of megakaryocytes without appreciable dysplasia. Immature CD34+ cellular elements corresponding to less than 1% of the marrow, without obvious fibrosis. Immunohistochemicals (PGM1, CD16) showed increased number of mast cells in the cytoplasm, in some of which nucleated rubella were observed. There was mild swelling of the interstitial web.

Treatment with corticosteroids and Immunoglobulin G (Octagam 10%, Octapharma) as rescue therapy and empirical antibiotic therapy with cefepime (Zefepime, Vocate) and vancomycin (Voxin, Vianex) for bacterial meningitis was started. Two days later, a new lumbar puncture was performed. CSF showed leukocytes at 10 cells/mm^3, glucose at

95 mg/dL (reference values 40–70 mg/dL) with a ratio of 58% (normal value above 50%), and protein at 109 mg/dL (reference values 15–45 mg/dL). Both the CSF culture and PCR were negative for bacterial or viral pathogens, including *CMV, VZV, HSV1/2, EBV, HHV, Enterovirus, Parechovirus, Escherichia coli k1, Haemophilus influenzae, Listeria monocytogenes, Neisseria meningitidis, Streptococcus agalactiae, Streptococcus pneumoniae,* and *Cryptococcus neoformans/gattii*.

A habit history of frequent spring water consumption reported by her closest contact, along with the reports of endemic tropical diseases on the island of her residency, raised the suspicion of leptospirosis infection, although the serological test of the first sample was negative. Based on that, eight days later, a second blood sample revealed positive IgM against *Leptospira* (immunochromatographic assay) and confirmed the diagnosis. Targeted therapy with 2 g of ceftriaxone intravenously, which was started empirically on the second day based on high grade of clinical suspicion was completed. On the 5th day, an attempt of analgosedation discontinuation was interrupted as the patient presented multiple episodes of myoclonus, exophoria, and impaired level of consciousness (GCS 6/15). A brain magnetic resonance imaging (MRI) revealed findings indicative of cytotoxic edema in the context of global hypoxic ischemic injury (Figure 1) of the caudate (white asterisk) and the lentiform (black asterisk) nuclei, bilaterally. On the corresponding apparent diffusion coefficient map (d), the same areas appeared hypointense.

Moreover, infratentorial leptomeningeal enhancement, most prevalent along the anterior aspect of the temporal lobes (arrows), was observed in axial T1-weighted MR images without (a and c) and after (b and d) administration of intravenous contrast. The findings were suggestive of the presence of meningitis/meningoencephalitis (Figure 2).

Despite targeted antibiotic therapy and multiple organ advanced supportive therapy, she presented no neurological improvement, remaining on a low level of consciousness and ventilator dependency. Furthermore, her hospitalization was complicated by multiple episodes of multidrug-resistant bloodstream infections, and ventilation-associated pneumonia, and ultimately the patients died two months later. Bloodstream infections were attributed to catheter-related infections and ventilator-associated pneumonias. The identified pathogens were *Pseudomonas aeruginosa* multidrug-resistant (MDR) and *Acinetobacter baumannii* MDR, as confirmed by positive blood cultures and bronchoalveolar lavage specimens. Further analysis revealed *Pseudomonas aeruginosa* resistance to β-lactams, quinolones, and carbapenems, while it exhibited sensitivity to colistin and aztreonam. *Acinetobacter baumannii*, on the other hand, demonstrated resistance to carbapenems, colistin, aminoglycosides, and ampicillin-sulbactam, with sensitivity noted to minocycline and intermediate sensitivity to tigecycline (MIC: 4 μg/mL). In response to these findings, targeted antibiotic therapy was administered based on antibiograms (colimycine Colistin Norma, tigecycline Tygacil Anfarm, ceftazidime Septax Vianex). Unfortunately, despite these efforts, the patient succumbed to multiorgan failure, attributed to multiple episodes of multidrug-resistant bloodstream infections leading to sepsis. The underlying cause of these recurring infections is believed to be associated with the patient's prolonged stay in the ICU, driven by ventilator dependency and a diminished level of consciousness following the initial insult of leptospirosis.

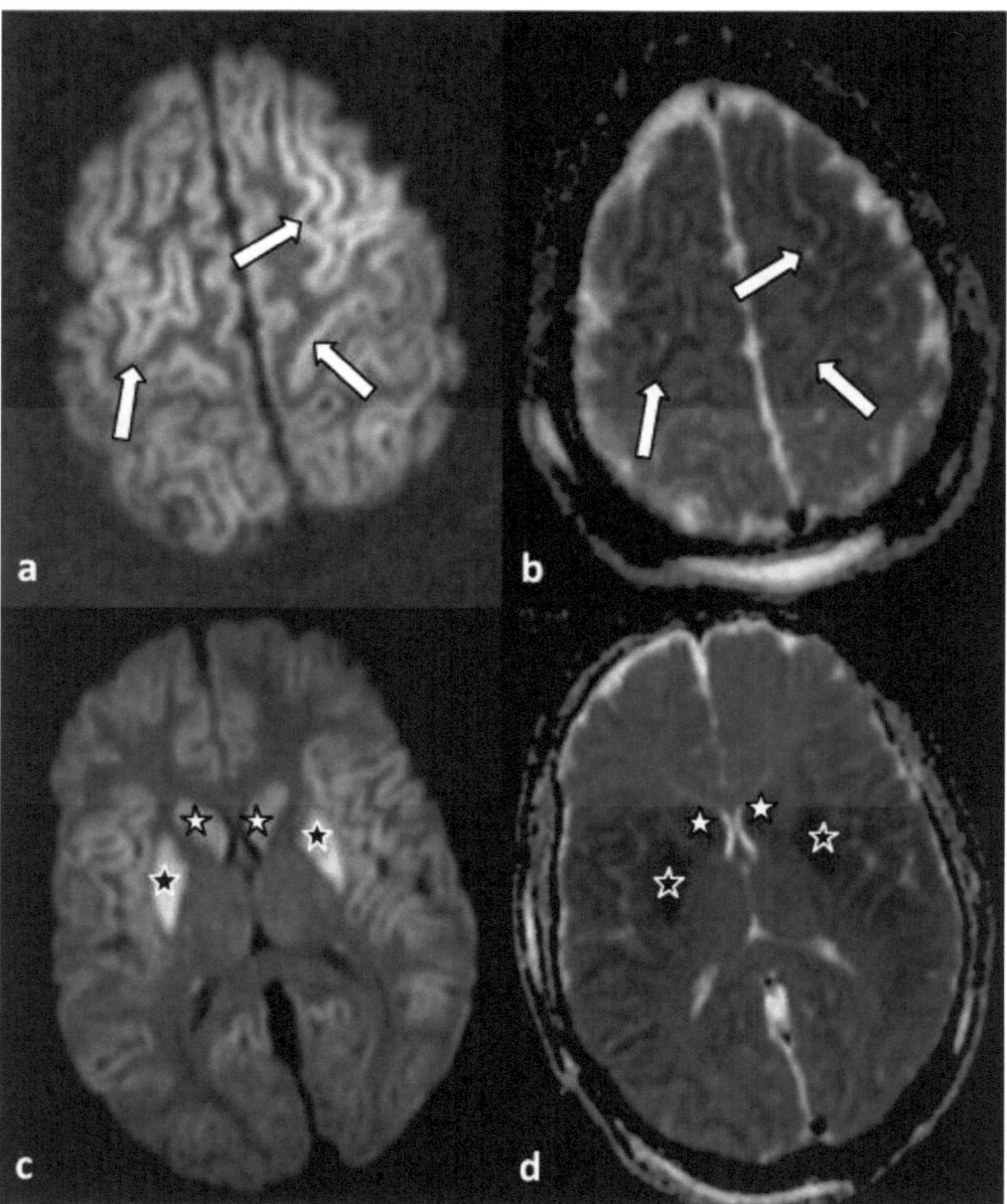

Figure 1. Axial diffusion-weighted imaging (**a**) and apparent diffusion coefficient map (**b**) at the level of the convexity, showing increased and decreased signal intensity of the cerebral cortex along both frontal lobes (arrows), respectively. Axial diffusion-weighted imaging (**c**) at the level of basal ganglia reveals symmetrical hyperintensity of the caudate (white asterisk) and lentiform (black asterisk) nuclei, bilaterally. On the corresponding apparent diffusion coefficient map (**d**), the same areas appear hypointense.

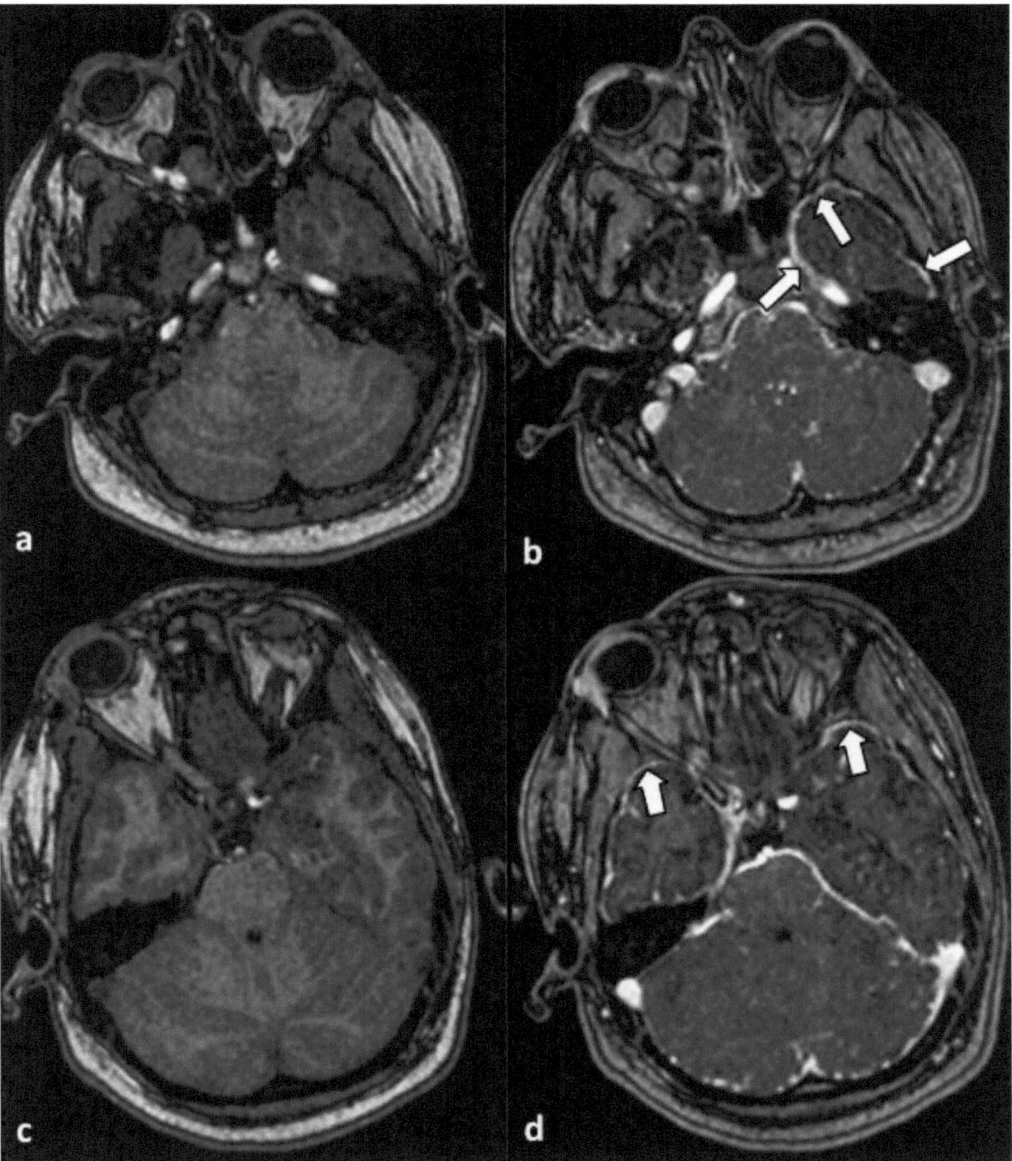

Figure 2. Axial T1-weighted MR images without (**a,c**) and after (**b,d**) administration of intravenous contrast material. An infratentorial leptomeningeal enhancement was noted, most prevalent along the anterior aspect of the temporal lobes (arrows). The findings were suggestive of the presence of meningitis/meningoencephalitis.

3. Discussion

Leptospirosis is a significant global health concern, substantiated by a 2017 Chinese study that documented a case-fatality ratio of 26.89 out of 7587 cases over a decade. Furthermore, Costa et al. approximated that there are 1.03 million cases of leptospirosis each year worldwide, contributing to an estimated 58,900 deaths. The authors also observed that the mortality rate of leptospirosis is equivalent to, or even surpasses, that of hemorrhagic fever in low-income and tropical countries. They concluded that leptospirosis is a primary cause of morbidity and mortality among zooanthroponotic diseases [4,9].

According to the Greek National Public Health Organization (GNPHO), in Greece, leptospirosis is a rare bacterial disease that affects approximately 20 individuals each year, resulting in an incidence rate of 0.13 to 0.31 per 100,000 population. However, the incidence rate may differ depending on the geographic region and season. It is important to note that Leptospirosis is likely underdiagnosed and underreported, which suggests that the actual incidence rate may be higher than the reported rate [10]. Recent studies conducted in southwestern Greece have estimated the incidence rate of Leptospirosis to be approximately 1.1 cases per 100,000 population in the area. The increased incidence rate may be attributed to climate change and the agricultural practices of the local population [11].

The clinical manifestation of the disease varies broadly from mild non-specific symptoms to multiple organ failure. Although the severe form of Weil's disease is rare, it can lead to life-threatening complications. The most common CNS manifestation is aseptic meningitis, accounting for 5% to 13% of all cases. Nevertheless, myelopathy, Guillain-Barre syndrome, meningoencephalitis, cerebellitis, cerebral hemorrhage, tremor neuralgia, facial palsy mononeuritis, movement disorders, and hemiplegia may also occur. Importantly, the clinical course of CNS in Weil's syndrome is usually associated with reversible neurological status [8]. The underestimation of leptospirosis mortality and morbidity rates in various countries is a topic of significant concern. Hartskeerl et al., have highlighted the absence of notification and epidemiological efforts as the primary reasons for this underestimation. Furthermore, the incidence rate of the disease is estimated only among individuals with severe leptospirosis around the world, leaving out those with milder cases. This exclusionary approach has resulted in a distorted perception of the actual incidence of the disease globally. The true extent of the impact of leptospirosis must be accurately documented and reported so that appropriate measures can be taken to address this health concern [12].

We present herein a case of Weil's syndrome associated with irreversible CNS disease. The presenting sign of the patient was coma, and she remained on a low conscious level over the clinical course. The combination of severe thrombocytopenia, altered mental status, and acute kidney injury raised the suspicion of possible thrombotic thrombopenic purpura (TTP), but the absence of schistocytes on peripheral blood smear excluded the diagnosis. The diagnosis of an infection, causing multiorgan failure attributed to disseminated intravascular coagulation (DIC) in combination with hypoperfusion seemed to be the most possible diagnosis. A thorough diagnostic process ruled out the most potential causes of coma, including common causes of bacterial meningitis, acute cerebrovascular accident, and thrombotic TTP with cerebral involvement. The positive serological test, combined with clinical data and environmental factors and the exclusion of other causes of coma, reinforced the diagnosis of leptospirosis with CNS involvement.

Coma as a presenting symptom in Weill's disease is uncommon. Only 10–15% of the patients may have a neurological symptom which often remains unrecognized [12,13]. In a small cohort of patients with leptospirosis with CNS involvement, altered sensorium and seizures have been reported as the most common neurological symptoms [14]. Two retrospective studies investigated the clinical characteristics in critically ill patients with severe leptospirosis. Samrot et al. reviewed 55 leptospirosis cases admitted to the ICU during 1998–2018 in tropical Australia. They reported no significant neurological signs except headache in 71% of hospital admissions [15]. Delmas et al. reported that a 4% of 134 consecutive leptospirosis cases presented with CNS involvement in the form of meningitis and encephalitis on admission. The mortality rate (identical for ICU, hospital mortality, and 28 d mortality) was 6.0% (95% CI, 2.6–11.4, eight patients) [16]. There are also a few case reports in the literature with CNS manifestation as a primary symptom of leptospirosis. All the patients suffered from headache, some of them also had symptoms such as vomiting, fever, and chills [14,17–20]. One patient had sudden onset of paraparesis, two had seizures, and one patient appeared with decreased responsiveness to commands, decreased verbal output, and inability to move his limbs [14,20–22]. Bandara et al. present two cases of neuroleptospirosis with headache, vomiting, and photophobia [23], and Zhang et al. reported a case of Leptospirosis-associated meningitis in a patient with sjögren's syndrome [24].

In a recent brief report from India, the authors analyzed seven consecutive patients with neuroleptospirosis admitted to a neurology ward. They had aseptic meningitis due to *Leptospira* without any systemic manifestation and they all recovered after antibiotic therapy with ceftriaxone and doxycycline [25].

In a study conducted in southwestern Greece among 45 patients with leptospirosis, only one patient presented CNS manifestations, specifically aseptic meningitis [11]. Neurological manifestations of leptospirosis are rare, and the most common is aseptic meningitis. The only report that we found in the literature that is similar to our case dates back to 2002 and involves a patient who presented with fever, coma, petechial rash, and conjunctival suffusion. The patient also had low PLTs and altered liver function. Leptospirosis was suspected, and penicillin and doxycycline were administered on day two despite the absence of laboratory evidence of leptospirosis. Serum IgM antibodies against *Leptospira* were negative, while IgG antibodies were positive. A four-fold increase in the titer of IgG antibodies confirmed the diagnosis one week later. After an extended stay in the ICU, the patient eventually passed away from a bloodstream infection [26]. In our case, our patient had negative IgM and IgG antibodies on the first evaluation upon admission, but after eight days the IgM antibodies were positive, confirming the diagnosis eventually. Although we started ceftriaxone on day two due to clinical suspicion, the patient died after two months in the ICU due to multiple episodes with multidrug resistant bloodstream infections and ventilator-associated pneumonia without any recovery from brain damage.

Although neuroleptospirosis is rare and coma even rarer, a history of risk exposure with symptoms such as headache, myalgia, jaundice, aseptic meningitis, and multiorgan failure will lead to the suspicion of leptospirosis, and appropriate diagnostic tests could confirm the diagnosis.

Diagnostic procedure includes direct methods of identifying the bacterium and indirect methods such as serological tests. Blood culture is the gold standard and has to be performed during the first week of the illness. Unfortunately, this is a demanding method with low diagnostic capability, useful to determine antibiotic sensitivity. PCR has to be performed in the first week, and shows high sensitivity and specificity. Serological methods detect antibodies by day six to ten of illness, and during their peak within three to four weeks. It is useful to measure antibodies with an interval of two weeks to compare them. This comparison has a high sensitivity and specificity [6].

In our case, the confounding factors of habitual spring water consumption, along with the reports of endemic tropical diseases on the island of her residency, raised the suspicion of leptospirosis infection, although the first serology was negative. Based on that, eight days later, a second blood sample revealed positive IgM against *Leptospira* (immunochromatographic assay) and confirmed the diagnosis.

The methodology used for the diagnosis of *Leptospira* was the GenBio IgM ImmunoDOT *Leptospira* test, which is a qualitative enzyme immunoassay that specifically detects IgM antibodies to *Leptospira biflexa* (serovar patoc 1). The test is intended for use in serum, plasma, heparinized whole blood, or finger-stick capillary blood. The microscopic agglutination test (MAT) is the preferred method, and is the current World Health Organization standard reference method [27]. The MAT method has high sensitivity and specificity, and permits the detection of group-specific antibodies. Despite its widespread application, the MAT method is constrained to highly specialized laboratories capable of maintaining live, hazardous stock serovar cultures. Criteria for laboratory diagnosis, as outlined by the Centers for Disease Control and Prevention (CDC), involve the isolation of leptospira from a clinical specimen, a significant four-fold or greater increase in *Leptospira* agglutination titer between acute and convalescent-phase specimens collected at intervals of greater than or equal to two weeks, or the visualization of *Leptospira* in a clinical specimen by immunofluorescence [28].

Presumptive diagnostic criteria are based on a leptospira agglutination titer equal to or exceeding 200 in single specimens from clinically symptomatic cases. Alternative methods for the detection of IgM antibodies during the acute phase, such as enzyme-linked microplate immunosorbent (ELISA) assays and an indirect hemagglutination (IHA) in vitro diagnostic procedure, are commercially available and reported to exhibit sensitivity and specificity comparable to the MAT method [29–31]. It is noteworthy that the MAT method has not been commercially distributed.

According to modified Faine's criteria for diagnosis of leptospirosis, our patient had a score of >25 (Part A, B, C/rapid test), which means that the diagnosis of leptospirosis is presumptive, with a sensitivity 89.39% and specificity of 58.82%, while the parts A + B + C /MAT $\geq$ 1800 and/or PCR had a sensitivity of 98.31% and specificity of 55.05 [30,31].

4. Conclusions

Leptospirosis remains a reemerging zooanthroponosis. Although CNS involvement does not appear to be the main presenting symptom, legionella still must be excluded in cases of aseptic meningitis with compatible epidemiological background. A high index of suspicion and a careful history of exposure is essential in order to consider leptospirosis as a possible diagnosis and start empirical treatment without waiting for the laboratory confirmation.

Author Contributions: C.A. and E.K.: conceptualization, writing, review and editing; A.P. and S.K.: data curation, writing, review and editing; I.K. and M.R.: data curation, writing. All authors have read and agreed to the published version of the manuscript.

Funding: This research received no external funding.

Institutional Review Board Statement: The study was conducted in accordance with the Declaration of Helsinki, and approved by the Institutional Ethics Committee of the University Hospital of Heraklion, Crete, Greece approved this publication. Approval number 42654. Date of approval protocol 19 December 2023.

Informed Consent Statement: Informed consent was obtained from the patient's father to publish this paper.

Data Availability Statement: Data are contained within the article.

Conflicts of Interest: The authors declare no conflict of interest.

References

1. Weil, A. Veber eine eigentümliche, mit milztumor, icterus und nephritis einhergehende, akute infektionskrankheit. *Dtsch. Arch. Klin. Med.* **1886**, *39*, 209.
2. Levett, P.N. Leptospirosis. *Clin. Microbiol. Rev.* **2001**, *14*, 296–326. [CrossRef]
3. World Health Organization. *Human Leptospirosis: Guidance for Diagnosis, Surveillance and Control*; No. WHO/CDS/CSR/EPH 2002.23; World Health Organization: Geneva, Switzerland, 2003.
4. Costa, F.; Hagan, J.E.; Calcagno, J.; Kane, M.; Torgerson, P.; Martinez-Silveira, M.S.; Stein, C.; Abela-Ridder, B.; Ko, A.I. Global Morbidity and Mortality of Leptospirosis: A Systematic Review. *PLoS Negl. Trop. Dis.* **2015**, *9*, e0003898. [CrossRef]
5. Harrison, N.A.; Fitzgerald, W.R. Leptospirosis—Can it be a sexually transmitted disease? *Postgrad. Med. J.* **1988**, *64*, 163–164. [CrossRef]
6. Rajapakse, S. Leptospirosis: Clinical aspects. *Clin. Med.* **2022**, *22*, 14–17. [CrossRef] [PubMed]
7. Turner, L.H. Leptospirosis I. *Trans. R. Soc. Trop. Med. Hyg.* **1967**, *61*, 842–855. [CrossRef] [PubMed]
8. Rajapakse, S.; Rodrigo, C.; Balaji, K.; Fernando, S.D. Atypical manifestations of leptospirosis. *Trans. R. Soc. Trop. Med. Hyg.* **2015**, *109*, 294–302. [CrossRef]
9. Yang, S.; Wu, J.; Ding, C.; Cui, Y.; Zhou, Y.; Li, Y.; Deng, M.; Wang, C.; Xu, K.; Ren, J.; et al. Epidemiological features of and changes in incidence of infectious diseases in China in the first decade after the SARS outbreak: An observational trend study. *Lancet Infect. Dis.* **2017**, *17*, 716–725. [CrossRef] [PubMed]
10. National Public Health Organization. Available online: https://eody.gov.gr/disease/leptospeirosi/ (accessed on 20 February 2024).

11. Gkentzi, D.; Lagadinou, M.; Bountouris, P.; Dimitrakopoulos, O.; Triantos, C.; Marangos, M.; Paliogianni, F.; Assimakopoulos, S.F. Epidemiology, clinical and laboratory findings of leptospirosis in Southwestern Greece. *Infect. Dis.* **2020**, *52*, 413–418. [CrossRef] [PubMed]
12. Hartskeerl, R.A.; Collares-Pereira, M.; AEllis, W.A. Emergence, control and re-emerging leptospirosis: Dynamics of infection in the changing world. *Clin. Microbiol. Infect.* **2011**, *17*, 494–501. [CrossRef] [PubMed]
13. Panicker, J.N.; Mammachan, R.; Jayakumar, R.V. Primary neuroleptospirosis. *Postgrad. Med. J.* **2001**, *77*, 589–590. [CrossRef]
14. Mathew, T.; Satishchandra, P.; Mahadevan, A.; Nagarathna, S.; Yasha, T.C.; Chandramukhi, A.; Subbakrishna, D.K.; Shankar, S.K. Neuroleptospirosis—Revisited: Experience from a tertiary care neurological centre from South India. *Indian. J. Med. Res.* **2006**, *124*, 155–162.
15. Samrot, A.V.; Sean, T.C.; Bhavya, K.S.; Sahithya, C.S.; Chan-Drasekaran, S.; Palanisamy, R.; Robinson, E.R.; Subbiah, S.K.; Mok, P.L. Leptospiral Infection, Pathogenesis and Its Diagnosis. A Review. *Pathogens* **2021**, *10*, 145. [CrossRef]
16. Delmas, B.; Jabot, J.; Chanareille, P.; Ferdynus, C.; Allyn, J.; Allou, N.; Raffray, L.; Gaüzere, B.-A.; Martinet, O.; Vandroux, D. Leptospirosis in ICU: A Retrospective Study of 134 Consecutive Admissions. *Crit. Care Med.* **2018**, *46*, 93–99. [CrossRef]
17. Özdemir, D.; Sencan, I.; Yıldirim, M.; Güçlü, E.; Yavuz, T.; Karabay, O. Andiscriminated aseptic meningitis case between rickettsia and leptospiral meningitis. *Eur. J. Gen. Med.* **2008**, *27*, 573. [CrossRef]
18. Waggoner, J.J.; Soda, E.A.; Seibert, R.; Grant, P.; Pinsky, B.A. Case report: Molecular detection of leptospira in two returned travelers: Higher bacterial load in cerebrospinal fluid versus serum or plasma. *Am. J. Trop. Med. Hyg.* **2015**, *93*, 238. [CrossRef]
19. Wang, N.; Han, Y.H.; Sung, J.Y.; Sen Lee, W.; Ou, T.Y. Atypical leptospirosis: An overlooked cause of aseptic meningitis. *BMC Res. Notes* **2016**, *9*, 16–19. [CrossRef] [PubMed]
20. Bhatt, M.; Rastogi, N.; Soneja, M.; Biswas, A. Uncommon manifestation of leptospirosis: A diagnostic challenge. *BMJ Case Rep.* **2018**, *2018*, bcr-2018. [CrossRef] [PubMed]
21. Chang, A.A.; Ranawaka, U.K.; Gunasekara, H.; Wijesekera, J.C. A case of primary neuroleptospirosis. *Ceylon Med. J.* **2003**, *48*, 143. [CrossRef] [PubMed]
22. Saeed, N.; Khoo, C.S.; Remli, R.; Law, Z.K.; Periyasamy, P.; Osman, S.S.; Tan, H.J. First reported case of neuroleptospirosis complicated with anton's syndrome. *Front. Neurol.* **2018**, *9*, 966. [CrossRef] [PubMed]
23. Bandara, A.G.N.M.K.; Kalaivarny, G.; Perera, N.; Indrakumar, J. Aseptic meningitis as the initial presentation of Leptospira borgpetersenii serovar Tarassovi: Two case reports and a literature review. *BMC Infect. Dis.* **2021**, *21*, 488. [CrossRef]
24. Zhang, Y.; Zheng, Y. Leptospirosis-associated meningitis in a patient with sjögren's syndrome: A case report. *BMC Infect. Dis.* **2023**, *23*, 778. [CrossRef]
25. Bismaya, K.; Dev, P.P.; Favas, T.T.; Pathak, A. Neuro-Leptospirosis: Experience from a tertiary center of North India. *Rev. Neurol.* **2023**, *3*, 238–243. [CrossRef]
26. Dimopoulou, I.; Politis, P.; Panagyiotakopoulos, G.; Moulopoulos, L.A.; Theodorakopoulou, M.; Bisirtzoglou, D.; Routsi, C.; Roussos, C. Leptospirosis presenting with encephalitis-induced coma. *Intensive Care Med.* **2002**, *28*, 1682. [CrossRef]
27. Turner, L.H. Leptospirosis II. *Trans. R. Soc. Trop. Med. Hyg.* **1968**, *62*, 880. [CrossRef]
28. Pappas, M.G.; Ballou, R.; Gray, M.R. Rapid serodiagnosis of leptospirosis using the IgM-specific dot ELISA: Comparison with the microscopic agglutination test. *Am. J. Trop. Med. Hyg.* **1985**, *34*, 346. [CrossRef] [PubMed]
29. Koo, D.; Wharton, M.; Birkhead, G. Case definitions for infectious conditions under Public Health Surveillance. *MMWR Recomm. Rep.* **1997**, *46*, 49.
30. World Health Organization. *Report of the First Meeting of the Leptospirosis Burden Epidemiology Reference Group*; WHO Press: Geneva, Switzerland, 2010.
31. Bandara, K.; Weerasekera, M.M.; Gunasekara, C.; Ranasinghe, N.; Marasinghe, C.; Fernando, N. Utility of modified Faine's criteria in diagnosis of leptospirosis. *BMC Infect. Dis.* **2016**, *16*, 446. [CrossRef] [PubMed]

Disclaimer/Publisher's Note: The statements, opinions and data contained in all publications are solely those of the individual author(s) and contributor(s) and not of MDPI and/or the editor(s). MDPI and/or the editor(s) disclaim responsibility for any injury to people or property resulting from any ideas, methods, instructions or products referred to in the content.

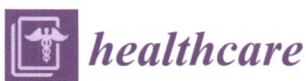

Review

Nursing Interventions for Client and Family Training in the Proper Use of Noninvasive Ventilation in the Transition from Hospital to Community: A Scoping Review

Jéssica Moura Gabirro Fernando [1], Margarida Maria Gaio Marçal [2], Óscar Ramos Ferreira [2,3], Cleoneide Oliveira [4], Larissa Pedreira [5] and Cristina Lavareda Baixinho [2,3,6,*]

1. Hospital Vila Franca de Xira, 2600-009 Vila Franca de Xira, Portugal; jessicafernando@esel.pt
2. Department of Fundamentals of Nursing, Escola Superior de Enfermagem de Lisboa, Nursing School of Lisbon, 1600-190 Lisbon, Portugal; margaridamarcal@campus.esel.pt (M.M.G.M.); oferreira@esel.pt (Ó.R.F.)
3. Nursing Research, Innovation and Development Centre of Lisbon (CIDNUR), 1900-160 Lisbon, Portugal
4. Medical School Estácio Idomed Quixadá, University Center Estacio do Ceará, Fortaleza 60035-111, Brazil; cleo_sbf@yahoo.com.br
5. Nursing School, Federal University of Bahia, Salvador 40170-110, Brazil; larissa.pedreira@uol.com.br
6. Center of Innovative Care and Health Technology (ciTechCare), 2414-016 Leiria, Portugal
* Correspondence: crbaixinho@esel.pt; Tel.: +35-19-33-254-269

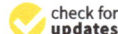

Citation: Fernando, J.M.G.; Marçal, M.M.G.; Ferreira, Ó.R.; Oliveira, C.; Pedreira, L.; Baixinho, C.L. Nursing Interventions for Client and Family Training in the Proper Use of Noninvasive Ventilation in the Transition from Hospital to Community: A Scoping Review. *Healthcare* 2024, 12, 545. https://doi.org/10.3390/healthcare12050545

Academic Editor: Christina Alexopoulou

Received: 10 January 2024
Revised: 17 February 2024
Accepted: 22 February 2024
Published: 25 February 2024

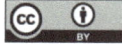

Copyright: © 2024 by the authors. Licensee MDPI, Basel, Switzerland. This article is an open access article distributed under the terms and conditions of the Creative Commons Attribution (CC BY) license (https://creativecommons.org/licenses/by/4.0/).

Abstract: Noninvasive ventilation is an increasingly disseminated therapeutic option, which is explained by increases in the prevalence of chronic respiratory diseases, life expectancy, and the effectiveness of this type of respiratory support. This literature review observes that upon returning home after hospital discharge, there are difficulties in adhering to and maintaining this therapy. The aim of this study is to identify nursing interventions for client and family training in the proper use of noninvasive ventilation in the transition from hospital to community. A scoping review was carried out by searching MEDLINE, CINAHL, Scopus, and Web of Science. The articles were selected by two independent reviewers by applying the predefined eligibility criteria. Regarding transitional care, the authors opted to include studies about interventions to train clients and families during hospital stay, hospital discharge, transition from hospital to home, and the first 30 days after returning home. The eight included publications allowed for identification of interventions related to masks or interfaces, prevention of complications associated with noninvasive ventilation, leakage control, maintenance and cleaning of ventilators and accessories, respiratory training, ventilator monitoring, communication, and behavioral strategies as transitional care priority interventions to guarantee proper training in the transition from hospital to community.

Keywords: noninvasive ventilation; transitional care; training; return home; discharge

1. Introduction

According to the Forum of International Respiratory Societies, respiratory diseases are one of the main causes of death and disability worldwide. One of the reasons for this is that 200 million people have chronic obstructive pulmonary disease (COPD), of whom approximately 3.2 million die every year. This problem is the third most frequent cause of death around the world. Additionally, asthma, one of the main chronic diseases, affects roughly 350 million people on the planet [1].

A research study involving 14,127 individuals ≥40 years of age with COPD observed that the 5-year mortality of COPD patients was 25.4% (29.9% in males and 19.1% in females). The mortality rate increased rapidly with age [2]. Furthermore, there are difficulties in the adherence to noninvasive ventilation (NIV) [3–5].

According to a 2020 report by the National Observatory of Respiratory Diseases, one of the activities offered by organizations for patients with respiratory disorders is related to promoting knowledge, information, and literacy in the different pathologies that are part of this category [2]. Consequently, and more specifically, it is crucial to educate and train clients to use NIV since there are individuals that need to continue its use after hospital discharge in order to promote care continuity, maintain their adherence to the treatment, and prevent worsening of the disease [1,3,5]. Not accomplishing these tasks implies the risk of going back to hospital.

The probability of developing several complications associated with NIV increases proportionally with its duration, client restlessness, and a constant need to adjust the mask [6]. Therefore, preventing complications by aiming for successful use of NIV is considered one of the main functions of nurses in the care of clients in critical situations who require NIV [6].

Complications related to the use of interfaces in NIV are the most frequent. They include discomfort caused by poor adjustment of masks and the pressure exerted by them (30% to 50% of cases); the feeling of claustrophobia (5% to 10%), which can trigger client restlessness; and pressure injuries, mostly in the nasal pyramid (5% to 10%). There are also complications related to pressure and air flow: dryness of oral and nasal mucosae (20% to 50%), nasal congestion (10% to 20%), and eye irritation resulting from leakage around the mask. Additionally, "gastric distention can also affect some clients, but it is rarely intolerable". Only 5% of clients showed more serious complications, such as aspiration pneumonia, hypotension, and pneumothorax [4].

Other causes for difficulties in adhering to the NIV are associated with non-acceptance of the need for domiciliary NIV, the fear of becoming "technology-dependent", and psychological issues such as anxiety and claustrophobia [5].

The initiation and maintenance of long-term home NIV represents a significant lifestyle change which intrinsically requires sustained effort on the part of the patient and often their family or caregivers [5], who usually mention difficulty in using NIV because of a lack of information that should be provided at hospital discharge [7].

The studies reinforce that patients and their caregivers show gaps in knowledge and insufficient skills to maintain NIV after discharge [8–10], which will affect the adherence and the capacity of the caregiver to provide care, with consequences such as insufficient functional improvement and unnecessary hospital readmissions [9,10].

These problems point out the need for a special intervention by health professionals, mainly nurses, oriented toward patients and family caregivers, not just because of the transition they are about to experience into the new role they will take on, but also to allow the possibility of obtaining better health results [10].

In order to minimize these issues, it is important to focus on coordination between hospitals and primary healthcare units, which should carry out prior assessments of the homes of the most critical patients before hospital discharge, including the possibility of evaluating the implementation of ventilation therapy [2].

The literature review performed by the authors observed that there are few studies on preparing people with NIV to return home and the strategies used to empower patients and families to return home. Nurses are the professionals who have responsibility for developing interventions in the area of education for the health of people under ventilation therapy that allow proper and safe transition from hospital to home. These procedures will help these clients and their relatives or other meaningful people to develop new cognitive and instrumental competencies that can effectively guarantee care continuity at home [8].

The objective of the present study was to identify nursing interventions for client and family training in the proper use of noninvasive ventilation in the transition from hospital to community.

2. Materials and Methods

2.1. Study Design

The method chosen was a scoping review. It allows for identification of the evidence types available on the subject, examination of study types, and detection and analysis of knowledge gaps [11]. An initial search identified several studies about nursing interventions oriented toward inpatients under NIV but found that studies addressing preparation to return home and transitional care of these patients are scarce.

The research question for the present review was formulated by applying the PCC (Population, Concept, Context) mnemonic [11]: What nursing interventions are implemented to train adult or elderly clients and family caregivers to use NIV at home after hospital discharge?

2.2. Eligibility Criteria

The object of study and the research question helped define the eligibility criteria of the studies to be included in this scoping review. To narrow the research strategy and increase the rigor and quality of the results, inclusion and exclusion criteria were defined for each of the elements of the PCC acronym, according to the methodology proposed by JBI [11] (Table 1).

Table 1. Eligibility criteria, Lisbon, 2023.

	Inclusion Criterion	Exclusion Criterion
P	Adults and elderly people submitted to NIV.	Age < 18 years.
C	Interventions to qualify clients and family caregivers to use and manage NIV: education and training, monitoring, communication, and behavioral strategies.	Interventions to qualify clients and families to use and manage IV. Formal caregivers.
C	Transitional care between hospital and community (hospital stay, hospital discharge, transition from hospital to home, first 30 days after returning home).	Residential facilities for elderly people, long-term care in health or social institutions, and rehabilitation units.

Regarding transitional care, the authors opted to include studies about interventions to train clients and family caregivers during hospital stay, hospital discharge, transition from hospital to home, and the first 30 days after returning home. This option is based on the concept of transitional care, which includes the notion that interventions to manage the transition from hospital to home can occur in three distinct steps: before clients leave the hospital, at hospital discharge, and between 48 h and 30 days after hospital discharge [10,12]. To be included in the sample, the articles had to address interventions in at least one of these phases, and their results had to allow for the identification of interventions that allow for training (client and family caregiver) on the use of noninvasive ventilation in the transition from hospital to community.

The chosen publication date period was from 2017 to 2023. This time frame is justified as we sought to obtain recent studies and considering that concern about transitional care is a recent development in healthcare [12]. A full text filter was applied, and only publications written in English or Portuguese were included. There was no restriction on the country of origin of the articles, only on the language used.

2.3. Data Collection

The search for publications was carried out in MEDLINE (via the PubMed platform), CINAHL, Scopus, and Web of Science databases (databases available at the university) by using terms in natural language and descriptors used in the indexing of each database. Table 2 shows the terms used in the search in the MEDLINE database.

Searches in the databases occurred in May 2023. Gray literature was also considered in the search, which included consulting Google Scholar and the Portuguese Open Access Scientific Repository. E-books, online handbooks, books, reports, dissertations, conference proceedings, documents from the ministry of health, general directorates of health, and available guidelines were accepted in this phase.

Table 2. Search strategy used in the MEDLINE database search (Lisbon, 2022).

	Search Strategy	Number of Articles
#1	((((((((((((((((((Elderl*(Title/Abstract))) OR (aged(Title/Abstract))) OR (age*(Title/Abstract))) OR (older person*(Title/Abstract))) OR (older adult*(Title/Abstract))) OR (middle age(Title/Abstract))) OR (younger adult(Title/Abstract))) OR (frail older adults(Title/Abstract))) OR (aged(MeSH Terms))) OR (frail elderly(MeSH Terms))) OR (adult, frail older(MeSH Terms))) OR (adults, frail older(MeSH Terms))) OR (adult, young(MeSH Terms))) OR (adults, young(MeSH Terms))) OR (middle age(MeSH Terms))) OR (middle aged(MeSH Terms))) NOT (children(MeSH Terms))) NOT (adolescent(MeSH Terms))) NOT (adolescence(MeSH Terms)))) Filters: Free full text, in the last 5 years	15,148
#2	((((((((((((((((((((Mechanical ventilator(Title/Abstract)) OR (Cpap ventilation Positive end expiratory pressures(Title/Abstract))) OR (Mechanical ventilation(Title/Abstract))) OR (Biphasic continuous positive airway pressure(Title/Abstract))) OR (Bilevel continuous positive airway pressure(Title/Abstract))) OR (Inspiratory positive pressure ventilation(Title/Abstract))) OR (Positive end expiratory pressure(Title/Abstract))) OR (Non-invasive ventilation(Title/Abstract))) OR (Noninvasive ventilation(Title/Abstract))) OR (NIV(Title/Abstract))) OR (BIPAP(Title/Abstract))) OR (CPAP(Title/Abstract))) OR (IPAP(Title/Abstract))) OR (EPAP(Title/Abstract))) OR (PEEP(Title/Abstract))) OR (Biphasic positive airway pressure(Title/Abstract))) OR (Continuous positive airway pressure(Title/Abstract))) OR (Non-invasive positive pressure ventilation(Title/Abstract))) OR (Artificial Ventilation(Title/Abstract))) OR (non invasive positive pressure ventilation(MeSH Terms))) OR (positive pressure non invasive ventilation(MeSH Terms)) Filters: Free full text, in the last 5 years	20,668
#3	(((((((transitional care(Title/Abstract)) OR (discharge(Title/Abstract))) OR (patient discharge(Title/Abstract))) OR (TCM(Title/Abstract))) OR (home nursing(Title/Abstract))) OR (discharge planning(MeSH Terms))) OR (discharge, patient(MeSH Terms))) OR (aides, home care(MeSH Terms)) Filters: Free full text, in the last 5 years	47,391
#4	(((((((intervention(Title/Abstract)) OR (capacitation(Title/Abstract))) OR (health education(Title/Abstract))) OR (information(Title/Abstract))) OR (early intervention education(MeSH Terms))) OR (habilitation(MeSH Terms))) OR (health education(MeSH Terms))Filters: Free full text, in the last 5 years	495,644
#5	#1 AND #2 AND #3 AND #4	148

In order to facilitate article organization and selection after the search process, the Rayyan® platform was used. Data screening and extraction was carried out independently by two researchers (JF and MM). When these researchers did not reach a consensus, a third researcher (CLB) was recruited to make the decision.

Documents obtained from the gray literature search that were not able to be uploaded to the software were digitized and analyzed independently by the 2 reviewers.

2.4. Data Processing and Analysis

The content extracted from the final bibliographic sample was entered into a Microsoft Excel table designed by the researchers and shared via cloud storage. It contained the following information: article title, author name(s), publication year, article type, objectives, methods, and main results/conclusions.

After extraction of results, a thematic synthesis was carried out to organize the interventions according to their nature.

A critical appraisal of the articles was not performed. The method does not oblige this evaluation. One of the peculiarities of this methodology is that it does not aim to analyze the methodological quality of the studies included, given that its objective, following the aforementioned, is not to find the best scientific evidence but rather to map the existing scientific evidence [11].

3. Results

In the first phase of the study, 220 articles were identified, of which 6 were duplicates. Reading titles and abstracts allowed the researchers to select 29 articles for full text reading. Application of the eligibility criteria to the articles available in the databases resulted in a set of six publications. Thirty-one documents were identified in the gray literature, of which two were included in the final sample (Figure 1).

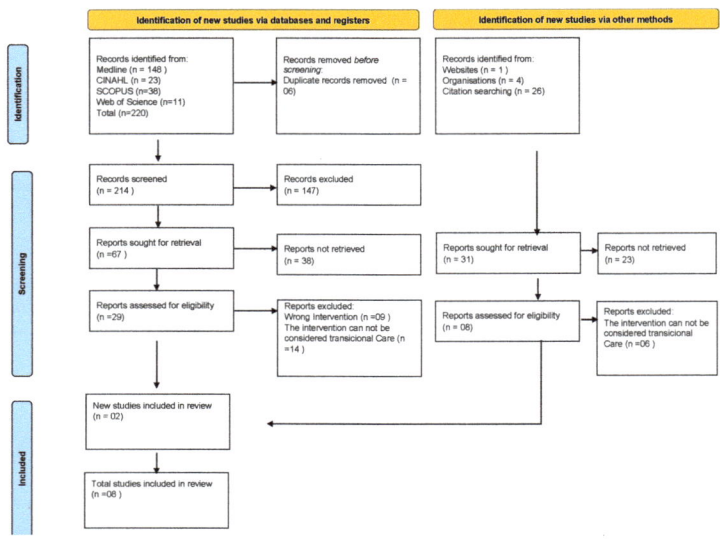

Figure 1. PRISMA-SR flowchart [13] (Lisbon, 2023).

Table 3 shows information about the eight documents selected in the present scoping review, such as objectives, document type, and results that answer the research question. The bibliographic sample was heterogeneous and included five literature reviews [9,14–17], a survey [18], a qualitative study [19], and a book [20]. Two documents were produced in Portugal [9,20], one in Spain [14], one in Germany [19], one in the United States [18], one in the England [15], one in China [16], and one in Brazil [17].

Table 3. Studies included in the scoping review (Lisbon, 2023).

Reference, Origin Country, and Publication Year	Study Design and Objectives	Results
[9] Portugal 2017	Integrative review	It is essential to define criteria for the care of people under NIV, including those for its prescription, maintenance, and evaluation. Equally fundamental are interface selection, initial setup, adjustments, and knowledge of NIV failure predictors. Noninvasive ventilation implies specific surveillance by clients, in which nurses play a prominent role.
[14] Spain 2017	Literature review. Identifying risk factors for incidence of skin injuries associated with clinical devices caused by NIV, preventive strategies to reduce them, and the most effective treatment for injuries that cannot be avoided.	The mask of choice was the facial one, and foam or hydrocolloid dressings were always applied on the nasal bridge. The condition of the skin under the interface and harness must be evaluated every 4 h (recommended) or every 11 h (maximum). The interface rotation strategy must be evaluated at 24 h if NIV is still needed on an ongoing basis.

Table 3. Cont.

Reference, Origin Country, and Publication Year	Study Design and Objectives	Results
[15] UK 2019	Systematic literature review. Evaluating the reason why clients needed long-term noninvasive positive pressure ventilation, describing some necessary nursing care procedures, and identifying some challenges experienced by nurses who provided home support when they interacted with these clients.	Noninvasive ventilation is a therapy that has been widely used in the home environment. Consequently, it is important that healthcare professionals understand the principles of its use in this setting and the challenges it can present for clients. Some crucial aspects that must be considered include the importance of proper mask adjustment, complications that clients can experience because of ventilation therapy, and how they can influence its effectiveness. Therefore, nurses are the professionals responsible for improving the way client care is managed at home by developing knowledge and specialized understanding of use of NIV in the domestic setting. This will promote client adherence, prevent complications, and decrease the number of hospital admissions. Using humidification units coupled to the ventilator can help some clients, but these units require daily cleaning. The container must be filled with boiled water so risk of contamination is reduced.
[18] United States 2019	Survey study. Collecting data about the experiences and care transition of clients, as well as factors associated with post-discharge follow-up.	There were inconsistencies in care transition processes. The authors recommended health education sessions, follow-up appointments, phone calls, and support for home care.
[19] Germany 2019	Qualitative study. Describing the quality of nursing care for clients submitted to NIV at home in Bavaria, Germany, and providing improvement recommendations from the perspective of health professionals.	This study described a heterogeneous and partly deficient care situation of people with NIV but showed that high quality care is possible if person-centered care is successfully implemented in all areas of service provision. Delivering person-centered care should be based on empowering ventilated patients to be completely involved in all decisions regarding their care and support. Care should support autonomy, focus on individuals' needs and preferences, and enable ventilated patients and their families to consider treatment options and make informed decisions. Successful person-centered care initially requires the appropriate attitude to meet people's needs (*outcomes and impact*), the involvement of ventilated patients in all decisions related to their care (*service delivery*), and a common vision of person-centered care provided by inspiring leadership (*vision and leadership*).
[16] China 2022	Literature review. Providing an overview of titration and follow-up of clients under noninvasive positive pressure ventilation. Focused on different technologies, modalities, managements, and cost-effectiveness used in Internet of Things-based telemonitoring of home mechanical ventilation.	Actively monitoring and communicating information during follow-up were crucial for long-term adherence. The medical Internet of Things will shift care from hospitals and clinics to homes and mobile devices. Patients may communicate with doctors or nurses at home via smart phones, mobile applications (apps), or the Internet. The Internet of Things allows users to access these "things" wherever and whenever they require them. There are a lot of opportunities for the Internet of Things to help remote caregivers ensure the safety of patients with noninvasive positive pressure ventilation and other wearable devices and raise warnings over critical situations. In this situation, providers should respond immediately to patient needs.
[17] Brazil 2022	Integrative review. Identifying the needs of critically ill patients who had to be submitted to NIV and their families, as well as nursing interventions that promoted adaptation of these patients and their families to NIV.	Adaptation of clients under NIV was promoted by implementing nursing interventions, both pharmacological and nonpharmacological. It is important to first adopt a nonpharmacological intervention, which includes four essential domains: communication, technology, comfort promotion, and environmental management. It is critical that nurses develop nursing technology competencies so that these professionals can allow technology and care to coexist harmoniously and develop activities oriented toward promoting clients' physical integrity.
[20] Portugal 2021	Book with evidence on COPD. Identifying nursing care that must be implemented to help clients with COPD regarding use of NIV during exacerbations and at home and informing them about the importance of motor and cardiorespiratory training for clients' activities of daily living with the purpose of maintaining their quality of life.	It is important to take a few breaks in the use of the mask for clients to moisten their face, humidify the oral mucosa, and clean the mouth with mouthwash. Some breathing techniques stood out, such as inhaling through the nose with the mouth closed, directing the air into the abdomen, carrying out diaphragmatic breathing, and slowly exhaling through the mouth with the lips half-closed. The study presented care procedures for different complications associated with NIV.

Of the studies identified, two refer to interventions carried out in hospital [14,19], three refer to interventions carried out at home [15,16,18], and three contain interventions covering the transactional period [9,17,20].

Analysis of the contents of the selected articles identified interventions related to masks or interfaces [13–15,17], prevention of complications associated with NIV [13,15,16,18–20], leakage control [15,20], maintenance and cleaning of ventilators and accessories [13,20], respiratory training [20], ventilator monitoring [13,16], and communication and behavioral strategies [17–20] (Table 4).

Table 4. Systematization of nursing interventions intended to train clients and family caregivers in correctly using NIV in the transition from hospital to community (Lisbon, 2023).

Nursing Interventions to Train Clients and Families to Correctly Use NIV in the Transition from Hospital to Community
Masks or interfaces [9,14,15,17,20] Teaching of mask or interface placement and training in their adjustment. - Full face masks: upper edge supported on the nose wings, lower edge resting on the chin. - Nose mask: resting on the nose wings between the nose and the upper lip. - First adjust the mask and then the harness, without exerting too much pressure.
Prevention of complications associated with NIV [9,14–17,20] Pressure injuries: - Correctly moisturize the skin. - Check the skin condition every two hours. - Use hydrocolloid or polyurethane dressings in the areas under highest pressure. - Remove the mask intermittently to provide the areas under highest pressure with some relief. Eye discomfort: - Apply artificial tears and wet eye dressings. Nasal congestion: - Wash the nose with saline solution. - Apply steroids and antihistamines. Dry mouth and nasal mucosae: - Clean the mouth with mouthwash. - Orally hydrate the mucosae by drinking liquids. - Use humidification units coupled to the ventilator (use boiled water to reduce risk of contamination). Abdominal distension: - Keep the mouth closed when using the NIV device. - Promote mobilization and elimination of secretions. - Use antiflatulents if necessary. - Do exercises that recruit the lower limbs. Risk of vomit aspiration: - Watch the clients for some time after they take solid and liquid food. - Keep clients in Fowler's position for at least 30 min after meals. - Remove the equipment in case of nausea or vomiting.
Leakage control [9,14,15,17,20] - Choose the mask correctly, opting for one with smaller dimensions, or change the mask type according to new needs and meet the requirements of each model. - During mask placement, make sure that it does not collide with the corners of the eyes and/or the mouth. - Observe the correct body position and make sure that the mask is placed when clients are in the proper position for receiving NIV. - Look around the mask in search of small leakages. - In case of the use of dental prosthesis, keep it in during the NIV procedure. - Avoid the presence of facial hair, namely beards. - Use fixation systems (for example, support for the chin).

Table 4. *Cont.*

Nursing Interventions to Train Clients and Families to Correctly Use NIV in the Transition from Hospital to Community
Maintenance and cleaning of ventilators and accessories [17,20] - Clean the external surface of the ventilator with a wet cloth. - Wash the filters once a month with warm water and soap, then dry them properly before inserting them again. It is essential to replace them every six months. - Disassemble the mask and accessories fully once a week, wash whatever possible with warm water and soap, and dry it properly before assembling it again. - Clean the circuit externally with a wet cloth, without using cleaning products. - Place the equipment on a flat and stable surface in an airy, low-humidity place. - Always have a spare mask and circuit.
Respiratory training [9,20] Instructing in and monitoring breathing techniques: - Inhale through the nose with the mouth closed, directing the air into the abdomen. - Carry out diaphragmatic breathing. - Slowly exhale through the mouth with the lips half-closed. Positions for relaxation and respiratory control: - Sitting: feet firmly touching the floor, body slightly tilted forward, and elbows resting on the thighs. - Lying down: right lateral decubitus with the headboard elevated. - Standing up: elbows resting on a surface (for instance a low wall, a counter), with the body slightly tilted forward. -Semi-Fowler's position. Techniques to clean the airway: - Inhale deeply. - Ensure proper hydration to guarantee secretion fluidification. - Carry out respiratory physical therapy. - Cough vigorously in one go, with the mouth open, to eliminate secretions.
Ventilator monitoring [9,14–16,19,20] - Reevaluate parameters up to three months after the beginning of the therapy. Subsequently, evaluation must occur annually. - Make sure the company that provided the equipment pays home visits at the beginning of the therapy and four weeks later. - Provide information about the presence of an alarm in the equipment, which allows identification of air leakage and consequent need to adjust the mask.
Communication and behavioral strategies [17–20] - Ensure a calm and quiet environment. - Speak in a soft and calm tone of voice. - Maintain eye contact with clients. - Keep a calm attitude, which conveys self-confidence and competence. - Promote resting and relaxation positions (for example, diaphragmatic breathing). - Learn how to put the mask on and attach it and do these procedures by yourself (if you are a client). - Provide information about the possible presence of alarms. - Suggest that clients try music therapy.

4. Discussion

The present scoping review gathered articles and gray literature material to answer the research question. Although research on NIV use has been fruitful over past years, the sample indicated that the studies about the topic were biomedically oriented and predominantly carried out in the hospital setting. Transitional care programs focused on training clients and families in the transition from hospital to home in order to guarantee adherence of the former to NIV were not identified.

Analysis of the articles showed mentions of interventions related to providing information to, training, and monitoring people so they could use and adapt to masks or interfaces [9,14,15,17], prevention of complications associated with NIV [9,15,16,18–20], leakage control [15,20], maintenance and cleaning of ventilators and accessories [9,20], respiratory training [16], ventilator monitoring [9,16], and communication and behavioral strategies [17–20] to promote continuous adherence to this therapy.

Transitional care programs centered on people who need to use NIV were not identified, which may contribute to the existing difficulties experienced by people in the community in terms of adhering to this therapy [20]. Since health systems aim to improve the quality of care delivered to clients, and consequently their experiences and clinical results, in order to minimize costs, it is urgent that care transitions between hospital and community be optimized for these patients.

Preparation, which must be initiated in the hospital, must include health education sessions, follow-up appointments, phone calls, and support for home care [10,20,21] with individualized care plans to fulfill clients' specific needs in order to minimize the chances of hospital readmission caused by worsening symptoms [15,16,21].

The discomfort and pressure caused by masks and the development of pressure injuries reinforce that crucial interventions should be part of the care plan, including guidance on correct mask adjustment, interface type switching, the choice of proper mask type and size, hygiene, skin hydration, and leakage control [9,14,15,17,19,20,22–25]. It is important to stress that, in addition to the quality of information provided to clients and their relatives, other factors affect treatment success, such as attention to comfort, pain control, collaboration with caregivers, and the quality of the relationship between healthcare professionals and clients/families [26].

A qualitative research study which interviewed 16 patients with chronic obstructive pulmonary disease (COPD) treated with NIV while hospitalized concluded that were some factors which promoted NIV tolerance, such as trust in the providers; a favorable impression of the facility and staff; understanding of why the mask was needed, how NIV works, and how long it will be needed; immediate relief of the threatening suffocating sensation; familiarity with similar treatments; use of meditation and mindfulness; and the realization that treatment was useful [27].

Studies also note that professionals need training and education concerning health issues related to the use of NIV [28,29] and how to educate and capacitate patients and their caregivers for the transition from hospital to community [10,12]; patients are more adherent with an intervention when they are involved in the decision-making process [30]. For these difficulties to be overcome, the authors proposed that the care plan be flexible enough to meet clients' individual needs and that there be a leader in the process who can train professionals so they can deliver safe care and ensure that multiprofessional teams have effective introduction, training, and supervision [19,20], for example, by discussing clinical cases [19], supporting family-centered care training, and making sure clients are treated with empathy and respect [19,20].

Empowering the patient with information and explanations regarding physiologic need and tangible benefits prior to initiating the device can establish a trusting relationship and reduce doubts and fears about this therapy [27,30], increasing adherence to the use of masks and interfaces and preventing complications associated with long-term maintenance [9,15,16,18–20,27,30]. Comfort of the intervention is dependent upon how well the patient and device work together for optimal physiologic outcomes [30].

Our results shows that leakage due to poor adjustment of the mask or inadequate fit with the patient's characteristics is a cause not only of nonadherence, but also of irritation and eye infections [15,20], which highlights the need for follow-ups with these patients at home for early detection of this problem and its complications. The discharge and transitional care plan includes a visit by the nurse in the first 2/3 days after discharge to assess the patient and the caregiver, their doubts and difficulties, and conditions at home [10], as well as precociously identify situations that pose a risk to adherence.

A consensus statement from the Agency for Clinical Innovation, that will be reviewed in 2024, observes that patients and caregivers should have a minimum level of skills and knowledge during acclimatization to NIV [31], namely about the maintenance and cleaning of ventilators and the changing or cleaning of filters and accessories such as humidifiers and nebulizers.

It should be noted that there are few studies on the follow-up of these patients at home and on interventions that can increase adherence to treatment and empower the patient to be independent in carrying out daily life activities. Future studies should explore this issue.

Another result from our SR concerns respiratory training with the aim of reducing dyspnea and consequent work of breathing, maintaining or improving tolerance to physical exercise, mobilizing secretions and assisting in their removal, and improving ventilation efficiency [20,30,31]. It is also important that these patients undergo muscle strengthening exercise training and activities of daily living training carried out with an energy compensation technique [30].

An aspect that did not emerge in the results, but that deserves attention in these patients who present a greater risk of falling [32], is the prevention of accidents. The transition plan and follow-up must provide for the assessment of risk factors, including environmental risk, advice on modifications, adaptation to space and equipment, and cognitive behavioral strategies that increase safety [10,32].

The results of the present scoping review allowed for verification that the main focus for clients in adherence to NIV should be on health education [9,11,14–16,18,19]. Given that nonadherence of clients to this practice results from lack of information, it is fundamental that nurses have sufficient scientific knowledge to formulate care plans that meet clients' needs regarding the use of NIV.

The aspects related to the relationship with the health team, communication, and behavioral strategies [17–20] indicated the need to speak in a soft and calm tone of voice and maintain visual contact and a calm attitude, which conveys self-confidence and competence, leading to clients feeling motivated to adhere to the treatment [25,33].

A study that had the objective of analyzing the impact of a brief psychological support intervention on adherence to NIV among patients with COPD concluded that the intervention group, which received cognitive behavioral therapy support, including counselling, relaxation, and mindfulness-based exercises, showed improvements regarding both adherence to NIV ($F(304) = 19.054$, $p < 0.001$) and quality of life ($F(156) = 10.264$, $p = 0.002$) after eight meetings compared to the control group. The results also showed a significant change in quality of life over time ($F(71.480) = 8.114$, $p = 0.006$) [33].

Future studies must explore the use of these strategies in improving adherence and training for clients and families so that they can be independent regarding NIV management, leading to improved self-care and execution of activities of daily living. Since the prevalence of people with NIV is high, and because it is estimated that prevalence will continue to increase as a result of the increasing prevalence of chronic respiratory diseases [9,19,20], as well as there being several difficulties with the use of masks and equipment and barriers to therapy continuity [5,7,8,14,15], it is recommended that transitional care programs to train clients and caregivers in NIV use be designed, implemented, and evaluated.

Resorting to e-health programs can improve communication between clients and professionals [1] and help clarify questions in a timely manner [34].

This study has limitations. The restriction on language and free access to full texts may have excluded articles that answered the research question and respected the eligibility criteria, allowing some articles to be excluded deductively, thus missing important results that may have contributed to answering the research question and formulating recommendations. Another limitation is the option of not evaluating the methodological quality of the included articles, which is accepted in the method but limits the evidence of the results and the recommendations for practice.

Despite these limitations, the results allow the authors to identify the existing nursing interventions aimed at training clients and families to correctly use NIV in the transition from hospital to community and also allow for the proposal of recommendations for future studies that should address the difficulties experienced by people and their families in transitioning from the hospital to the community. Given the little evidence available on interventions in this period, qualitative studies are recommended [35] to bring attention to the voices of these people and their families to help identify strategies to focus care and allow adherence to NIV.

5. Conclusions

Hospital discharge planning must be initiated during hospital stay and aim to identify clients' and family caregivers' needs so they are met at home. For this goal to be achieved, it is necessary to implement several nursing interventions related to health education, specifically to necessary precautions concerning mask adjustment, equipment handling, prevention or resolution of complications that may emerge during the process, respiratory training, and cognitive behavioral strategies oriented toward reducing anxiety and clarifying questions, which are common issues for most NIV users.

As a recommendation for clinical practice, the authors suggest continuing education of healthcare professionals. It is also important and necessary to inform multiprofessional teams about the presence of schematic and visual supporting materials intended to improve dissemination of practical information for the final objective of improving quality of care delivered to patients submitted to NIV, thus promoting greater adherence to using this type of therapy at home.

Additionally, the present review points out the need to design new studies on transitional care programs that impact correct use of NIV at home.

Author Contributions: Conceptualization, J.M.G.F., M.M.G.M., and C.L.B.; methodology, Ó.R.F., L.P., C.O., and C.L.B.; software, J.M.G.F., M.M.G.M., and C.L.B.; validation, Ó.R.F., L.P., C.O., and C.L.B.; formal analysis, Ó.R.F. and C.L.B.; investigation, J.M.G.F., M.M.G.M., L.P., C.O., Ó.R.F., and C.L.B.; resources, C.L.B.; data curation, C.L.B. and Ó.R.F.; writing—original draft preparation, J.M.G.F., M.M.G.M., L.P., C.O., Ó.R.F., and C.L.B.; writing—review and editing, J.M.G.F., M.M.G.M., L.P., C.O., Ó.R.F., and C.L.B.; visualization, J.M.G.F., M.M.G.M., L.P., C.O., and C.L.B.; supervision, C.L.B. and Ó.R.F.; project administration, C.L.B. and Ó.R.F.; funding acquisition, C.L.B. and Ó.R.F. All authors have read and agreed to the published version of the manuscript.

Funding: The present study was funded by the Center for Research, Innovation, and Development in Nursing in Portugal by means of grants provided to some of the authors (CIDNUR, Psafe2transition_2021).

Institutional Review Board Statement: Not applicable.

Informed Consent Statement: Not applicable.

Data Availability Statement: The original contributions presented in the study are included in the article, and further inquiries can be directed to the corresponding author.

Conflicts of Interest: The authors declare that this research was conducted in the absence of any commercial or financial relationships that could be construed as a potential conflict of interest.

References

1. Forum of International Respiratory Societies. The Global Impact of Respiratory Disease, 3rd ed.; European Respiratory Society. 2021. Available online: https://firsnet.org/images/publications/FIRS_Master_09202021.pdf (accessed on 22 September 2023).
2. Park, S.C.; Kim, D.W.; Park, E.C.; Shin, C.S.; Rhee, C.K.; Kang, Y.A.; Kim, Y.S. Mortality of patients with chronic obstructive pulmonary disease: A nationwide populationbased cohort study. *Korean J. Intern. Med.* **2019**, *34*, 1272–1278. [CrossRef] [PubMed]
3. Le Bouar, G.; Boyer, D.; Artaud-Macari, E.; Molano, L.C.; Viacroze, C.; Cuvelier, A.; Patout, M. Noninvasive ventilation (NIV) adherence for chronic respiratory failure treatment. *Eur. Respir. J.* **2018**, *52* (Suppl. S62), PA2376. [CrossRef]
4. Gupta, S.; Ramasubban, S.; Dixit, S.; Mishra, R.; Zirpe, K.G.; Khilnani, G.C.; Khatib, K.I.; Dobariya, J.; Marwah, V.; Jog, S.A.; et al. ISCCM Guidelines for the Use of Non-invasive Ventilation in Acute Respiratory Failure in Adult ICUs. *Indian J. Crit. Care Med.* **2020**, *24* (Suppl. S1), S61–S81. [CrossRef] [PubMed]
5. Spurr, L. The treatment burden of long-term home noninvasive ventilation. *Breathe* **2021**, *17*, 200291. [CrossRef] [PubMed]
6. Davidson, A.C.; Banham, S.; Elliott, M.; Kennedy, D.; Gelder, C.; Glossop, A.; Church, A.C.; Creagh-Brown, B.; Dodd, J.W.; Felton, T.; et al. BTS/ICS guideline for the ventilatory management of acute hypercapnic respiratory failure in adults. *Thorax* **2016**, *71*, ii1–ii35. [CrossRef] [PubMed]

7. Hess, D.R. Noninvasive Ventilation for Acute Respiratory Failure. *Respir. Care* **2013**, *58*, 950–972. [CrossRef]
8. Ferreira, S.; Nogueira, C.; Conde, S.; Taveira, N. Ventilação não-invasiva. *Rev. Port. Pneumol.* **2009**, *15*, 655–677. Available online: https://www.redalyc.org/pdf/1697/169718537006.pdf (accessed on 22 September 2023). [CrossRef]
9. Pinto, C.; Sousa, P. Ventilação não invasiva: Uma revisão integrativa da literatura. In *Construindo Conhecimento em Enfermagem à Pessoa em Situação Crítica*; Dixe, L.M., Sousa, P., Gaspareiria, P., Eds.; Instituto Politécnico de Leiria: Leiria, Portugal, 2017; pp. 89–104. Available online: http://hdl.handle.net/10400.8/2882 (accessed on 22 May 2023).
10. Ferreira, B.A.d.S.; Gomes, T.J.B.; Baixinho, C.R.S.L.; Ferreira, M.R. Transitional care to caregivers of dependent older people: An integrative literature review. *Rev. Bras. Enferm.* **2020**, *73*, e20200394. [CrossRef]
11. Munn, Z.; Peters, M.D.J.; Stern, C.; Tufanaru, C.; McArthur, A.; Aromataris, E. Systematic Review or Scoping Review? Guidance for Authors When Choosing between a Systematic or Scoping Review Approach. *BMC Med. Res. Methodol.* **2018**, *18*, 143. [CrossRef] [PubMed]
12. Menezes, T.M.d.O.; de Oliveira, A.L.B.; Santos, L.B.; de Freitas, R.A.; Pedreira, L.C.; Veras, S.M.C.B. Hospital transition care for the elderly: An integrative review. *Rev. Bras. Enferm.* **2019**, *72* (Suppl. S2), 294–301. [CrossRef] [PubMed]
13. Tricco, A.C.; Lillie, E.; Zarin, W.; O'Brien, K.K.; Colquhoun, H.; Levac, D.; Moher, D.; Peters, M.D.J.; Horsley, T.; Weeks, L.; et al. PRISMA Extension for Scoping Reviews (PRISMA-ScR): Checklist and Explanation. *Ann. Intern. Med.* **2018**, *169*, 467–473. [CrossRef]
14. Raurell-Torredà, M.; Romero-Collado, A.; Rodríguez-Palma, M.; Farrés-Tarafa, M.; Martí, J.; Hurtado-Pardos, B.; Florencio, L.P.-S.; Saez-Paredes, P.; Esquinas, A. Prevención y tratamiento de las lesiones cutáneas asociadas a la ventilación mecánica no invasiva. Recomendaciones de expertos. *Enferm Intensiva.* **2017**, *28*, 31–41. [CrossRef]
15. Rolfe, S. Non-invasive positive pressure ventilation in the home setting. *Br. J. Community Nurs.* **2019**, *24*, 102–109. [CrossRef]
16. Jiang, W.P.; Wang, L.; Song, Y.L. Titration and follow-up for home noninvasive positive pressure ventilation in chronic obstructive pulmonary disease: The potential role of tele-monitoring and the Internet of things. *Clin. Respir. J.* **2021**, *15*, 705–715. [CrossRef] [PubMed]
17. Rio, A.S.P.C.; Ramos, F.A.M. Promotion the critically ill patient adaptation to noninvasive ventilation: An integrative literature review. *BJHR* **2022**, *5*, 21878–21899. [CrossRef]
18. Jones, B.; James, P.; Vijayasiri, G.; Li, Y.; Bozaan, D.; Okammor, N.; Hendee, K.; Jenq, G. Patient Perspectives on Care Transitions From Hospital to Home. *JAMA Netw. Open* **2022**, *5*, e2210774. [CrossRef]
19. Klingshirn, H.; Gerken, L.; Hofmann, K.; Heuschmann, P.U.; Haas, K.; Schutzmeier, M.; Brandstetter, L.; Ahnert, J.; Wurmb, T.; Kippnich, M.; et al. How to improve the quality of care for people on home mechanical ventilation from the perspective of healthcare professionals: A qualitative study. *BMC Health Serv. Res.* **2021**, *21*, 1–14. [CrossRef] [PubMed]
20. Cordeiro, M.C.O. *DPOC: Abordagem a 360° do Hospital para o Domicílio*; Lusodidacta: Sintra, Portugal, 2021.
21. Klingshirn, H.; Gerken, L.; Hofmann, K.; Heuschmann, P.U.; Haas, K.; Schutzmeier, M.; Brandstetter, L.; Wurmb, T.; Kippnich, M.; Reuschenbach, B. Comparing the quality of care for long-term ventilated individuals at home versus in shared living communities: A convergent parallel mixed-methods study. *BMC Nurs.* **2022**, *21*, 224. [CrossRef] [PubMed]
22. Pierucci, P.; Portacci, A.; Carpagnano, G.E.; Banfi, P.; Crimi, C.; Misseri, G.; Gregoretti, C. The right interface for the right patient in noninvasive ventilation: A systematic review. *Expert Rev. Respir. Med.* **2022**, *16*, 931–944. [CrossRef] [PubMed]
23. Fidalgo Fernandes, A.F.; Romão da Veiga Branco, M.A. Interdependent nursing interventions as sensitive indicators of quality—Care in noninvasive mechanical ventilation. *Millenium J. Educ. Technol. Health* **2023**, *2*, e28233. [CrossRef]
24. Shikama, M.; Nakagami, G.; Noguchi, H.; Mori, T.; Sanada, H. Development of Personalized Fitting Device with 3-Dimensional Solution for Prevention of NIV Oronasal Mask-Related Pressure Ulcers. *Respir. Care* **2018**, *63*, 1024–1032. [CrossRef]
25. Perry, M.A.; Jones, B.; Jenkins, M.; Devan, H.; Neill, A.; Ingham, T. Health System Factors Affecting the Experience of Non-Invasive Ventilation Provision of People with Neuromuscular Disorders in New Zealand. *Int. J. Environ. Res. Public Health* **2023**, *20*, 4758. [CrossRef]
26. D'orazio, A.; Dragonetti, A.; Campagnola, G.; Garza, C.; Bert, F.; Frigerio, S. Patient Compliance to Non-Invasive Ventilation in Sub-Intensive Care Unit: An Observational Study. *J. Crit. Care Nurs.* **2018**, *11*, e65300. [CrossRef]
27. McCormick, J.L.; Clark, T.A.; Shea, C.M.; Hess, D.R.; Lindenauer, P.K.; Hill, N.S.; Allen, C.E.; Farmer, M.S.; Hughes, A.M.; Steingrub, J.S.; et al. Exploring the Patient Experience with Noninvasive Ventilation: A Human-Centered Design Analysis to Inform Planning for Better Tolerance. *Chronic Obstr. Pulm. Dis.* **2022**, *9*, 80–94. [CrossRef]
28. Elena, B.; Tommaso, P.; Gianluca, F.; Mario, S.; Antonello, N. The importance of education and training for noninvasive ventilation: Suggestions from the literature. *Egypt. J. Intern. Med.* **2019**, *31*, 435–441. [CrossRef]
29. Alqahtani, J.S.; AlAhmari, M.D. Evidence based synthesis for prevention of noninvasive ventilation related facial pressure ulcers. *Saudi Med. J.* **2018**, *39*, 443–452. [CrossRef] [PubMed]
30. Strickland, S.L. The Patient Experience During Noninvasive Respiratory Support. *Respir. Care* **2019**, *64*, 689–700. [CrossRef] [PubMed]
31. NSW Agency for Clinical Innovation. *Domiciliary Non-Invasive Ventilation in Adult Patients*; A Consensus Statement; ACI: Sydney, NSW, Australia, 2012.
32. Baixinho, C.L.; Bernardes, R.A.; Henriques, M.A. How to evaluate the risk of falls in institutionalized elderly people. *Rev. Baiana Enferm.* **2020**, *34*, e34861. [CrossRef]

33. Volpato, E.; Banfi, P.; Pagnini, F.P. Promoting Acceptance and Adherence to Noninvasive Ventilation in Chronic Obstructive Pulmonary Disease: A Randomized Controlled Trial. *Psychosom. Med.* **2022**, *84*, 488–504. [CrossRef] [PubMed]
34. Jiang, W.; Song, Y. Internet of things-based home noninvasive ventilation in COPD patients with hypercapnic chronic respiratory failure: Study protocol for a randomized controlled trial. *Trials* **2022**, *23*, 393. [CrossRef] [PubMed]
35. de Oliveira, E.S.F.; Baixinho, C.L.; Presado, M.H.C.V. Qualitative research in health: A reflective approach. *Rev. Bras. Enferm.* **2019**, *72*, 830–831. [CrossRef] [PubMed]

Disclaimer/Publisher's Note: The statements, opinions and data contained in all publications are solely those of the individual author(s) and contributor(s) and not of MDPI and/or the editor(s). MDPI and/or the editor(s) disclaim responsibility for any injury to people or property resulting from any ideas, methods, instructions or products referred to in the content.

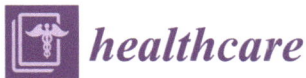

Article

Reduction in the Incidence Density of Pressure Injuries in Intensive Care Units after Advance Preventive Protocols

Ru-Yu Lien [1,2], Chien-Ying Wang [3,4,5,6], Shih-Hsin Hung [1,2,7], Shu-Fen Lu [1,2], Wen-Ju Yang [1], Shu-I Chin [1], Dung-Hung Chiang [4,5], Hui-Chen Lin [8], Chun-Gu Cheng [3,9,10,11,*] and Chun-An Cheng [3,12,*]

1. Department of Nursing, Taipei Veterans General Hospital, Taipei 112201, Taiwan; rylien@vghtpe.gov.tw (R.-Y.L.); hungsh@vghtpe.gov.tw (S.-H.H.); sflu@vghtpe.gov.tw (S.-F.L.); wjyang2@vghtpe.gov.tw (W.-J.Y.); sichin@vghtpe.gov.tw (S.-I.C.)
2. School of Nursing, National Yang Ming Chiao Tung University, Taipei 112304, Taiwan
3. Department of Exercise and Health Sciences, University of Taipei, Taipei 111036, Taiwan; wangcy@vghtpe.gov.tw
4. School of Medicine, National Yang Ming Chiao Tung University, Taipei 112304, Taiwan; dhchiang2@vghtpe.gov.tw
5. Department of Critical Care Medicine, Taipei Veterans General Hospital, Taipei 112201, Taiwan
6. Division of Trauma, Department of Emergency Medicine, Taipei Veterans General Hospital, Taipei 112201, Taiwan
7. Department of Nursing, Chang Jung Christian University, Tainan 711301, Taiwan
8. School of Nursing, College of Nursing, Taipei Medical University, Taipei 11031, Taiwan; cecilia@tmu.edu.tw
9. Department of Emergency Medicine, Taoyuan Armed Forces General Hospital, Taoyuan 32549, Taiwan
10. Department of Emergency Medicine, Tri-Service General Hospital, National Defense Medical Center, Taipei 11490, Taiwan
11. Department of Emergency, Wan Fang Hospital, Taipei Medical University, Taipei 11696, Taiwan
12. Department of Neurology, Tri-Service General Hospital, National Defense Medical Center, Taipei 11490, Taiwan

* Correspondence: er08@aftygh.gov.tw (C.-G.C.); cca@ndmctsgh.edu.tw (C.-A.C.); Tel.: +886-3-4801-604 (C.-G.C.); +886-2-8792-7173 (C.-A.C.)

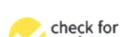

Citation: Lien, R.-Y.; Wang, C.-Y.; Hung, S.-H.; Lu, S-F.; Yang, W.-J.; Chin, S.-I.; Chiang, D.-H.; Lin, H.-C.; Cheng, C.-G.; Cheng, C.-A. Reduction in the Incidence Density of Pressure Injuries in Intensive Care Units after Advance Preventive Protocols. *Healthcare* 2023, *11*, 2116. https://doi.org/10.3390/healthcare11152116

Academic Editors: Paolo Cotogni and Christina Alexopoulou

Received: 18 June 2023
Revised: 8 July 2023
Accepted: 21 July 2023
Published: 25 July 2023

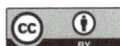

Copyright: © 2023 by the authors. Licensee MDPI, Basel, Switzerland. This article is an open access article distributed under the terms and conditions of the Creative Commons Attribution (CC BY) license (https://creativecommons.org/licenses/by/4.0/).

Abstract: (1) Background: Patients who are critically ill or undergo major surgery are admitted to intensive care units (ICUs). Prolonged immobilization is the most likely cause of pressure injuries (PrIs) in the ICU. Previous studies of Western populations found that effective protocols could reduce the incidence of PrIs, and the efficacy of systemic targeted intervention protocols in preventing PrIs in the Chinese population needs to be surveyed. (2) Methods: We reviewed cases of PrIs in the ICUs of Taipei Veterans General Hospital from 2014 to 2019. The ICU nurses at the hospital began to implement targeted interventions in January 2017. The incidence density of PrIs was calculated by dividing the number of PrIs by person days of hospitalizations in the pre-bundle (2014–2016) and post-bundle (2017–2019) stages. Poisson regression was performed to compare the trend of incidence densities. (3) Results: The incidence density of PrIs was 9.37/1000 person days during the pre-bundle stage and 1.85/1000 person days during the post-bundle stage ($p < 0.001$). The relative risk (RR) was 0.197 (95% confidence interval: 0.149–0.26). The incidence densities of iatrogenic PrIs and non-iatrogenic PrIs decreased as the RRs decreased. (4) Conclusions: Targeted interventions could significantly reduce the incidence of PrIs. Healthcare providers must follow the bundle care protocol for PrI prevention to improve the quality of healthcare and promote patient health.

Keywords: pressure injury; bundle care; incidence density reduction

1. Introduction

Pressure injuries (PrIs) are areas of skin, and possibly tissue, that have been damaged by continuous pressure on specific body prominence areas. They are common adverse events in intensive care units (ICUs), and the majority of PrIs are preventable [1]. Patients who are admitted to ICUs with critical illnesses are often immobile and require bed rest;

as a result, they are potentially prone to experiencing edema due to a poor venous return, circulation dysfunction, and hemodynamic instability with vasopressors. Some patients suffered from respiratory failure and required mechanical ventilation, agitation and required restraints, and exposure to moisture due to incontinence. The risk factors for PrIs are advanced age and obesity; the risk of PrIs increases as age and weight increase [2]. The incidence of adult PrIs ranges from 12% to 33% [3,4]. PrIs have significant impacts on patients, including pain, restricted mobility, wound infection, and psychological burden. They reduce quality of life and increase the risk of complications, resulting in longer hospital stays and increased health care costs [5].

The best way to prevent PrIs is to maintain clean and dry skin, avoid prolonged durations in the same position, and ensure the appropriateness of padding and mattresses to alleviate pressure. If PrIs are detected, prompt cleaning and management of the affected area should be undertaken in addition to necessary treatment. Due to the severity and complexity of their illnesses, critically ill patients are subjected to prolonged immobilization, have insufficient perfusion and poor nutritional statuses, and are at a higher risk for developing PrIs than general ward patients. Preventive interventions for PrIs focus on multiple factors and require the combination of various strategies to achieve optimal results. There was an association between the reduced risk of PrIs and preventive interventions, and bundle care is based on noteworthy, evidence-based interventions [6].

There are some care measures for and evidence on the prevention of PrIs. However, the implementation of prevention strategies is often not optimal [3,4]. Standard bundle care for PrI prevention can enable healthcare providers to control modifiable risk factors and enhance the quality of nursing care [7]. Previous studies have shown that the use of care bundles for skin care, including silicone dressing, skin protectants, comprehensive skin assessments from head to toe, heel offloading, the early identification of pressure sources, and repositioning, can effectively prevent PrIs by reducing the incidence density of PrIs [8–10]. The SSKIN (surface, skin investigation, kinetics/keep moving, incontinence/moisture, and nutrition/hydration) Care Bundle has been used frequently [11]. Previous studies found that the SSKIN bundle could effectively reduce the incidence of PrIs, improve patient outcomes, and enhance nurse compliance [12,13].

The main priority for nurses who administer critical care is the preservation of life quality during the treatment of life-threatening conditions rather than PrI prevention. Nurses with a heavy load take care of critical patients by monitoring vital signs and alerting physicians to life-threatening situations and have paid less attention to PrI prevention in the past. PrI prevention is an important issue of healthcare quality. Evidence-based critical care is necessary to prevent PrIs in the ICU. We used retrospective data from tertiary teaching hospitals in northern Taiwan before and after bundle care to evaluate the effect of PrI prevention to assess whether the trend of PrI incidence reduced.

The aim of this study was to evaluate the efficacy of care bundle use in PrI prevention by considering the influence on the incidence density of PrIs compared with the pre-bundle stage. Standardized and regular bundle care bundles for PrI prevention are designed by multidisciplinary teams to reduce PrI incidence and promote patient health. Such teams provide evidence on the benefits of care bundles for PrI prevention in the critical care setting.

2. Materials and Methods

2.1. Materials and Methods

This study was a review of the clinical data of adult ICU patients in Taipei Veterans General Hospital; there were 42 beds in the ICUs. The ICUs were the medical ICU and the surgical ICU. This study was a retrospective observation case–control study; the data were obtained from the nursing information system. The patients were hospitalized in ICUs from 1 January 2014 to 31 December 2019, in one medical center in northern Taiwan. The exclusion criteria were patients who underwent cardiac catheterization, and patients who were younger than 18 years of age. The patients that received cardiac catheterization on schedule had milder illnesses, and those younger than 18 years old had complex conditions. Data on sex, age, length of stay, body weight, comorbidities, disease severity, and use of sedatives, muscle relaxants, or inotropic agents were collected from the information system of ICUs.

The team who implemented bundle care for PrIs included critical care physicians, critical care nurses, wound care specialist nurses, and a member of the medical quality team who developed the SSKIN Care Bundle based on evidence in the literature [11]. Every patient who was admitted to ICUs was assessed by using the Braden Scale to determine their risk for PrIs [14], and high-risk patients were assigned to air suspension bed because the surface was supported with protection. The patients were repositioned every 2 hours and encouraged to move early, and the angle of their head did not exceed 30 degrees. To protect the urine or stool from irritating the skin, water was used for cleaning and the skin was kept dry. The nutrition evaluation was performed during hospitalization and twice every week to assess the patients' intake of protein and calories. The items of the SSKIN care bundle are shown in Table 1. PrIs were defined by the European Pressure Ulcer Advisory Panel (EPUAP) and the National Pressure Ulcer Advisory Panel (NPUAP). A PrI is localized damage to the skin and/or underlying tissue, typically occurring over bony prominences, resulting from pressure with or without shear. Incidence density was calculated by dividing the number of new cases of PrIs by the total patient days of hospitalizations in the ICUs.

Table 1. The items and actions of SSKIN bundle care of pressure injuries' prevention.

Items	Action
Surface	Air suspension bed for patients with higher risk of pressure injuries. The others use a pressure-reduced bed. When lying flat, place a pillow under both knees and calves to keep the heels off the bed. When lying on the side, place a pillow (at a 30-degree angle) behind the back to relieve pressure on the coccyx. The shoulder and hip joints on the side should be slightly tilted outward to relieve pressure. Bend the leg on the upper side, place a pillow between the knees, and ensure that the knees are not under pressure and the ankles are elevated. After turning over, adjust the position of the head and place a rolled towel behind the ear. Artificial skin pressure reduction products should be used at the pressure points when using a nasal intermittent positive pressure ventilation and loosened every 2 hours to inspect the skin. Ensure nasogastric tube or endotracheal tube fixed with Ω sharp without stressing nasal wings, and oxygen mask without pressuring nasal bridges or auricles with foam dressings.
Skin investigation	New patients and during reposition period, a real-time "head-to-toe" assessment of overall skin temperature, color, moisture status, and integrity, with particular attention to bony prominences. During each shift period, the overall risk for pressure injuries was assessed using the Braden Scale [1], which includes factors such as sensory perception, moisture, activity, mobility, nutrition, and friction/shear. A score of ≤14 is used to identify patients at high risk for pressure injuries. Check that the tubes are not under pressure by skin. Avoid compressing area that includes redness and refrain from massaging bony prominences.

Table 1. *Cont.*

Items	Action
Kinetics/keep moving	The turning schedule and prohibited actions were strictly followed to assist in changing the patient's position and limb placement correctly every 2 h. Encourage early movement, perform physical therapy, relieve spasticity, and limit sedative use. The bed should be leveled before turning the patient, and grasp the turning sheet closer to the patient's side and lift, avoiding pushing or pulling. After turning over, raise the foot end of the bed before elevating the head end, ensuring that the angle does not exceed 30 degrees and replace the position of the pulse oximeter.
Incontinence/moisture	Identify the stage of incontinence-associated dermatitis and fungal infection. Cleanse the skin affected by incontinence with water. To protect irritable skin from the urine or stool, keep skin clean and dry.
Nutrition/hydration	The nutritionists evaluated each patient after hospitalization and assessed their nutritional statuses twice every week to ensure adequate intake of protein and calories.

The care bundle for PrI prevention has been used in routine nursing care in critical care units since 1 January 2017. The care bundle for PrI care and prevention included good training and education before 2017. During the implementation phase, the nurse leader assessed the care bundle weekly to ensure compliance. Approximately 90% of nurses use the bundle. The primary outcome was the incidence density of PrIs. This study was approved by the Institutional Review Board (TPEVGH_IRB number: 2020-07-002CC on 24 June 2020).

2.2. Statistical Analysis

The distribution of categorical variables was analyzed using chi-square tests, while independent t tests were assessed for continuous data. Regarding exposure and nonexposure case numbers summed with an alpha of 0.05 and power of 80%, 1547 in each group and a total of 3094 was required. The periods were divided into two groups based on the time before (2014–2016) and after the implementation (2017–2019) of the target bundle care intervention. Poisson regression with log-linear regression for count data was performed to compare the incidence densities between two periods of all PrIs and different types of PrIs. $p < 0.05$ was considered to indicate a significant difference. The statistical analysis was performed using SPSS version 21.0 software.

3. Results

There were 4538 patients who were hospitalized in ICUs and data on a total of 64,171 patient day hospitalizations were obtained from the clinical information system. After excluding patients younger than age 18 and patients who received cardiac catheters (258 patients and 1031 patient day hospitalizations), the total number of patients was 4280 patients along with 63,140 patient day hospitalizations. The incidence density of PrIs was 9.37/1000 person days before the implementation of bundle care, and the incidence density of PrIs was 1.85/1000 person days after the implementation ($p < 0.001$) (Figure 1). The number of patients who required restraints in the ICU was significantly decreased. There were insignificant differences in sex, age, comorbidities, disease severity score, various laboratory values, and use of analgesics, sedatives, or vasopressors between the two stages (Table 2).

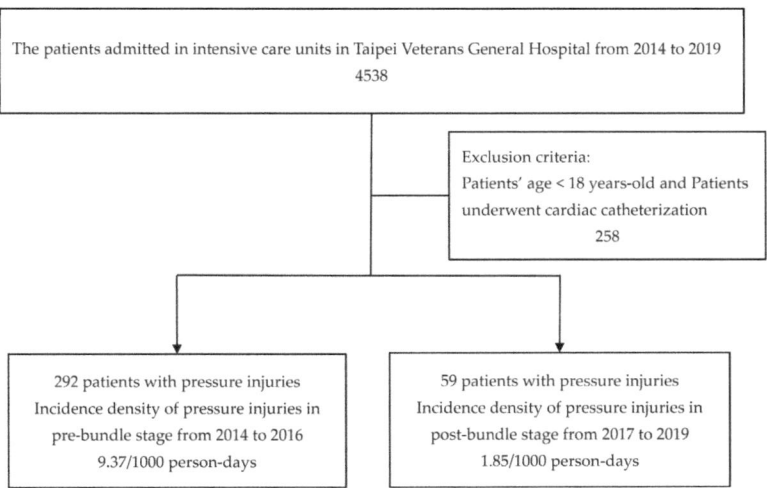

Figure 1. Flow chart of this study.

Table 2. Comparison of control variables between the two periods.

Variables	Pre-Bundle Stage (n = 2134)	Post-Bundle Stage (n = 2146)	p
The cases of PrIs	292	59	<0.001 *
Incidence density (/1000 person days) of PrIs	9.37	1.85	<0.001 *
Sex (Male)	1356 (63.54%)	1345 (62.67%)	0.539
Age	67.18 ± 17.53	67.55 ± 15.98	0.839
Length of stay	14.60 ± 11.52	14.90 ± 12.55	0.555
Glasgow Coma scale	10.84 ± 4.111	10.88 ± 3.927	0.805
Body weight	62.86 ± 14.57	63.48 ± 14.83	0.179
Albumin (g/dL)	2.886 ± 0.597	3.100 ± 0.592	0.214
Ventilation	8.422 ± 7.466	8.205 ± 7.800	0.419
Potassium (mEq/L)	3.977 ± 0.813	3.921 ± 0.718	0.407
Sodium (mEq/L)	139.8 ± 7.491	140.3 ± 7.272	0.694
Calorie achievement rate	72.57 ± 21.19	69.37 ± 22.48	0.722
Charlson comorbidity index	5.29 ± 2.32	5.02 ± 2.27	0.184
APACHE II score within first day	21.20 ± 7.03	22.32 ± 8.36	0.169
APACHE II score	20.21 ± 7.58	19.75 ± 8.45	0.175
Pain scores	1.64 ± 1.52	1.49 ± 1.96	0.360
Incontinence-associated dermatitis	447 (20.95%)	462 (21.53%)	0.642
Restraints	1908 (89.41%)	1871 (87.19%)	0.024 *
Sedation	1410 (66.07%)	1473 (68.64%)	0.073
Muscle relaxant	32 (1.5%)	31 (1.44%)	0.881
Inotropic agents	368 (17.24%)	372 (17.33%)	0.938
Pain control	1651 (77.37%)	1669 (77.78%)	0.75
Ventilation	1944 (91.1%)	1931 (89.98%)	0.213
Life support system	115 (5.39%)	112 (5.22%)	0.804
Nurse–patient ratio	2.53 (0.01)	2.6 (0.02)	0.374

* $p < 0.05$; PrIs: pressure injuries; APACHE II score: Acute Physiology and Chronic Health Evaluation II score. Life support system included Extracorporeal Membrane Oxygenation, Intra-Aortic Balloon Pump, and Continuous Venous Hemofiltration.

Before the implementation of the care bundle, the highest incidence density of PrIs in the ICU was 11.16 episodes/1000 person days during 2015. However, the comprehensive implementation of the SSKIN care bundle began in 2017, and the incidence density significantly decreased to 2.37 episodes/1000 person days in 2017 and reached the lowest of 1.24 episodes/1000 person days in 2019. There was a significant reduction of 88.89% in the incidence density of PrIs between 2015 and 2019 (Figure 2).

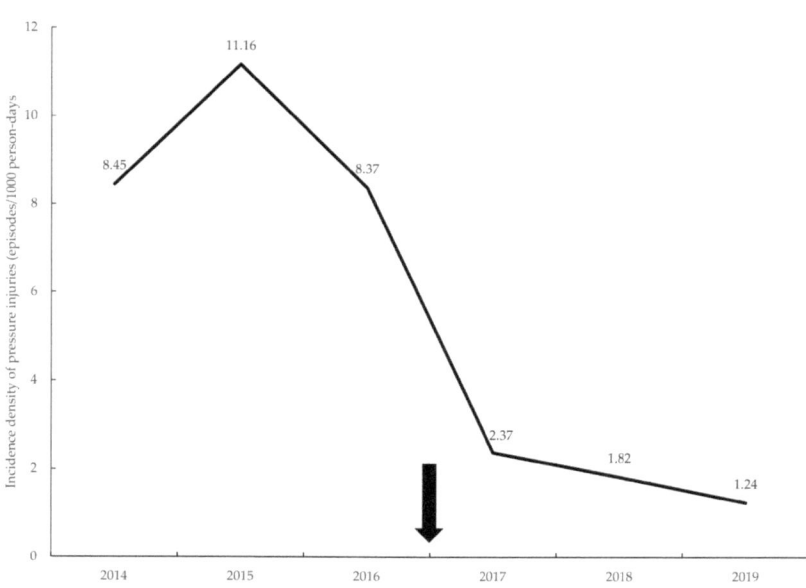

Figure 2. The incidence density of pressure injury in intensive care units. Bundle care implemented since 2017 (arrow).

The sacrum was the most common site of non-iatrogenic PrIs in the ICU before the implementation of the care bundle, followed by the ischial area and heels. The nose was the most common site of iatrogenic PrIs in the ICU, followed by the auricle in pre-bundle stage (Supplementary Table S1. The cases of different sites existing in iatrogenic and non-iatrogenic pressure injuries). The cases of iatrogenic and non-iatrogenic PrIs were significantly reduced after bundle care (Figure 3). The incidence density of non-iatrogenic PrIs significantly decreased from 6.67 to 0.84 episodes/1000 person days, with an RR of 0.126 (95% C.I.: 0.085–0.189, $p < 0.001$). The incidence density of iatrogenic PrIs significantly decreased from 2.7 to 1 episode/1000 person days, with an RR of 0.371 (95% C.I.: 0.247–0.558, $p < 0.001$) (Table 3).

The incidence density of PrIs in the ischium was the most significantly decreased, from 1.44 to 0.03 episodes/1000 person days with an RR of 0.022 (95% C.I.: 0.003–0.157, $p < 0.001$), and from 2.5 to 0.41 episodes/1000 person days with an RR of 0.162 (95% C.I.: 0.09–0.292, $p < 0.001$) in the sacrum as well as from 2.12 to 0.25 episodes/1000 person days with an RR of 0.118 (95% C.I.: 0.057–0.246, $p = 0.001$) in the lower limbs, but the reduction was not significant from 0.42 to 0.16 episodes/1000 person days with an RR of 0.375 (95% C.I.: 0.134–1.051, $p = 0.062$) in the back. The incidence density of PrIs in the nasal bridges was the most significantly decreased, from 0.55 to 0.06 episodes/1000 person days with an RR of 0.115 (95% C.I.: 0.026–0.496, $p = 0.004$); from 0.51 to 0.13 episodes/1000 person days with an RR of 0.244 (95% C.I.: 0.081–0.729, $p = 0.012$) in the face; and from 0.67 to 0.25 episodes/1000 person days with an RR of 0.371 (95% C.I.: 0.164–0.838, $p = 0.017$) in the auricle, but the reduction was not significant in the nasal wings, from 0.67 to 0.41 episodes/1000 person days with an RR of 0.603 (95% C.I.: 0.302–1.205, $p = 0.152$), and in the upper limbs, from 0.29 to 0.16 episodes/1000 person days with an RR of 0.541 (95% C.I.: 0.181–1.615, $p = 0.271$) (Table 3).

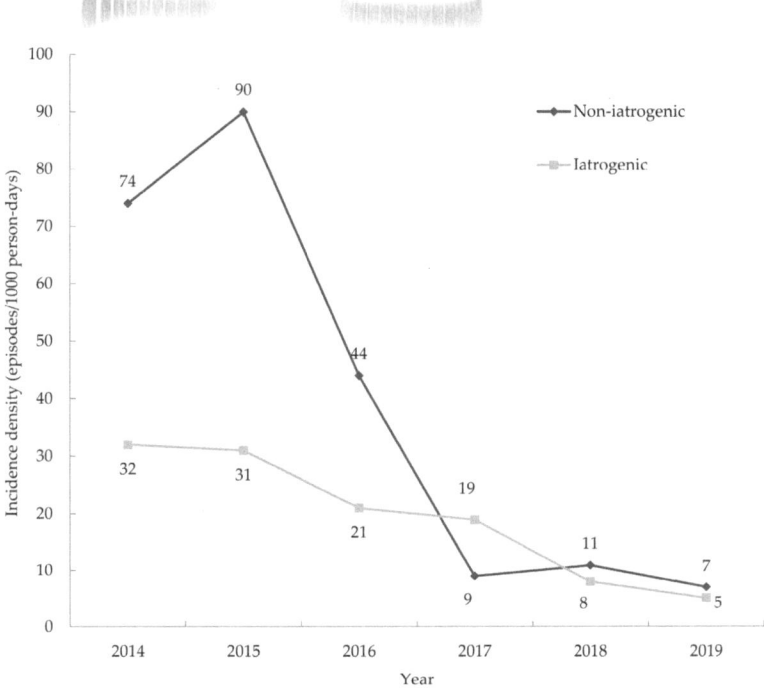

Figure 3. Cases of non-iatrogenic and iatrogenic pressure injuries in intensive care units.

Table 3. The incidence density and relative risk of different types of pressure injuries before and after care bundle implementation.

	Pre-Bundle Stage Incidence Density (/00)	Post-Bundle Stage Incidence Density (/00)	Relative Risk	p
Overall PrIs	9.37	1.85	0.197 (95% C.I.: 0.149–0.26)	<0.001 *
Non-iatrogenic PrIs	6.67	0.84	0.126 (95% C.I.: 0.085–0.189)	<0.001 *
Sacrum	2.5	0.41	0.162 (95% C.I.: 0.09–0.292)	<0.001 *
Back	0.42	0.16	0.375 (95% C.I.: 0.134–1.051)	0.062
Ischium	1.44	0.03	0.022 (95% C.I.: 0.003–0.157)	<0.001 *
Occiput	0.19	0		
Low limbs	2.12	0.25	0.118 (95% C.I.: 0.057–0.246)	0.001 *
Knee	0.35	0.03	0.089 (95% C.I.: 0.011–0.686)	0.02 *
Ankle	0.45	0.13	0.278 (95% C.I.: 0.092–0.846)	0.024 *
Heel	1.32	0.09	0.071 (95% C.I.: 0.022–0.23)	<0.001 *
Iatrogenic PrIs	2.7	1	0.371 (95% C.I.: 0.247–0.558)	<0.001 *
Nose	1.22	0.47	0.385 (95% C.I.: 0.212–0.699)	0.002 *
Nasal wings	0.67	0.41	0.603 (95% C.I.: 0.302–1.205)	0.152
Nasal bridge	0.55	0.06	0.115 (95% C.I.: 0.026–0.496)	0.004 *
Auricle	0.67	0.25	0.371 (95% C.I.: 0.164–0.838)	0.017 *
Face	0.51	0.13	0.244 (95% C.I.: 0.081–0.729)	0.012 *
Upper limbs	0.29	0.16	0.541 (95% C.I.: 0.181–1.615)	0.271

* $p < 0.05$. PrIs: pressure injuries; 95% C.I.: 95% confidence interval.

4. Discussion

This study found that the incidence of PrIs was significantly reduced after the implementation of care bundle intervention for 3 years. It was a new intervention with systemic prevention compared to previous routine nurse care in the Chinese population. In the long term, healthcare workers can fully understand the benefit of such measures that are designed to promote patient health by reducing the incidence of PrIs. Care bundles are essential to clinical practice. Although the overall iatrogenic and non- iatrogenic PrIs were decreased, there was still no significant reduction in the back, upper limbs, and nasal wings. They need more aggressive methods to reduce their incidence.

A recent study showed that integrating PrI prevention into practice significantly reduced the incidence of hospital-acquired PrIs (HAPI). The number of HAPI cases decreased from nine to one from the pre-intervention to post-intervention periods [15]. A prospective intervention using a prevention bundle was implemented in another study, and it significantly reduced the cumulative incidence rate of medical-device-related PrIs by 90% [16]. In our study, the number of PrI cases decreased from 121 to 12 (in 2015 vs. in 2019), resulting in a 90% reduction. A previous study found a significant reduction in the cumulative incidence density of PrIs in an intervention based on evidence-based skin care compared to the control group ($p = 0.04$, 18.1% vs. 30.4%) [17]. Another study observed a decrease in the incidence density of acquired PrIs from 15.5% before the intervention to 2.1% after the preventive intervention supported by wound ostomy continence nurses [9]. In our study, following the implementation of the care bundle, the incidence density of PrIs decreased from 9.37 to 1.85 episodes/1000 person days ($p < 0.001$), indicating that the care bundle for PrI prevention effectively reduces the occurrence of PrIs.

A multidisciplinary clinical and risk assessment team intervened for PrI prevention and used the SSKIN bundle care for PrI prevention. They found a reduction in the incidence of HAPI from 6.1‰ to 1.1‰, representing an 83.5% decrease [18]. Our study showed a similar finding, with a decrease of 80.26% of deceased patients. It emphasized that all patients should undergo a risk assessment within 2 h of admission and every 8 h thereafter. Furthermore, high-risk patients should be placed on pressure-relieving mattresses, undergo position changes at least every 2 h, and receive support to improve their nutritional status. For patients at a high risk, preventive dressings (sacrum, heels, hips) should be used to reduce the incidence of PrIs in critically ill patients [19]. Our check time in every shift time was approximately 8 h, and there was a reduction in the incidence of PrIs when compared with the pre-intervention stage. Nutritional status should be evaluated after ICU admission by a nutritionist and twice every week during the ICU stay. The care bundle was established by a multidisciplinary team incorporating evidence-based knowledge and implemented in clinical practice for PrI prevention. The results enhanced the effectiveness of prevention efforts in overall PrIs and iatrogenic and non-iatrogenic PrIs.

Before the intervention, the most common sites of iatrogenic PrIs were the auricle and nasal wings, followed by the nasal bridge (Supplementary Table S1: The cases of different sites of non-iatrogenic and iatrogenic pressure injuries). After the implementation of the care bundle, the nasal wings were still the most common site with an insignificant reduction. Patients undergoing oral or gastrointestinal surgery or swallowing difficulties need nasal–gastric tubes, and endotracheal tubes from the nose or mouth inserted for respiratory failure must be properly fixed in the philtrum area, leading to persistent PrIs in the nasal wings. We added foam padding to the inner edge of the nasal wings beginning in 2018, and the number of PrIs in the nasal wings decreased from 2018 to 2019. We addressed PrIs caused by oxygen masks by increasing the length of foam padding and using more effective materials.

The main sites of PrIs were peripheral oxygen saturation monitors and splints (two cases). This potentially results in nursing staff, with a busy clinical workload, failing to adequately reposition finger-type oxygen saturation monitors after turning the patient. Ring-type oxygen saturation monitors replaced the finger-type monitors for patients with poor peripheral circulation after discussions with the monitor team and administrators and timely repositioning of the finger-type monitors. The close inspection of the skin condition at the bony prominence area was performed when removing the splint in a timely manner during each shift time, and foam padding was implemented to prevent PrIs caused by splints.

The most common sites of non-iatrogenic PrIs were the sacrum, followed by the ischium and heel before the care bundle intervention. After the care bundle intervention, PrIs in the ischium and heel were almost completely prevented. It emphasizes relieving pressure on vulnerable areas and bony prominences in any position and elevating the head of the bed while not exceeding 30 degrees. PrIs in the sacrum still existed with five sacral PrIs annually, which need more strategies to address. This potentially resulted from a higher acuity and severity of illness in ICU patients and some self-mobilized patients with an inadequate maintenance of the 30-degree positioning of pillows.

There was an insignificant reduction in incidence density in the back, nasal wings, and upper limbs. The potential reason was the maintenance of 26 °C in the public units to save electronic energy based on a government policy that caused the patients' back to easily sweat when lying for a long duration. The colder temperature of air conditions could be set to reduce patients' sweating. Because an air suspension bed is used for patients with a higher PrI risk, some patients with an intermittent risk may progressively develop PrIs. The wide usage of air suspension in ICUs could reduce the incidence of PrIs in the future. A nasogastric tube and endotracheal tube were fixed on nasal wings in the emergency room or general rooms before transfer to ICUs, and new technology needs to be promoted to other units of the hospital to further reduce the PrIs in nasal wings. In addition, the gastrectomy encouraged for long-term nasal–gastric feeding could reduce PrIs in nasal wings. The majority of intravenous injections and artery lines were performed in the upper limbs, while careful repositioning was needed to prevent compression and early change to a central-line insertion in the subclavian or femoral veins to reduce PrIs in the upper limbs. In addition, a smart clothing study to prevent PrIs is ongoing [20]. Although albumin insignificantly increased (2.89 to 3.1 g/dL), trend nutrition improved after frequent nutritionist support for patients in the ICUs.

The liability profile could be excluded by proper documentation of the adequacy of the precautionary measures [21]. Many interventions for PrIs may only be effective in the short term [6], and our study showed persistent effectiveness for 3 years. The care bundle intervention proposed in this study is an effective approach for preventing PrIs in critically ill patients. Furthermore, this study brought about significant policy changes by only shifting from the traditional practice of repositioning every 2 hours (left side, right side, supine) to a concept of integrated intervention avoiding pressure on specific sites. At the initial implementation of the care bundle in the clinical practice of critical care, there was some resistance due to the increased workload by changing existing beliefs and habits with significant pushback. Through continuous communication with interdisciplinary collaboration to focus on the directions of enhancing patients' safety and improving the quality of healthcare, colleagues gradually became more accepting of changing their beliefs. The knowledge and skills regarding the care bundle were consistently taught during on-the-job training and prevocational education. The psychometric properties of the Pressure Ulcer Management Self-Efficacy Scale of nurses related to the care of PrIs in Taiwan [22] were included. A balanced distribution of nurses would improve the quality of care for PrIs [23]. Bundle care could be successful based on a nursing team designed with consulting expertise, reducing the barriers to promoting standard forms of care into regular care with good education and feedback audits to establish nursing facilities for the care of PrIs [13].

There are some limitations in our study. First, this study utilized a retrospective review of electronic health records. There were some missing or incomplete data due to various reasons, and the incidence density of PrIs may be underestimated. Second, there was a trend change in this study rather than a direct causal relationship between the care bundle and the reduction in the incidence density of PrIs. Third, the severity of PrIs was not surveyed. Fourth, the IRB granted approval for a retrospective study before 2020, and the incidence density persistently decreased by 1.2, 0.4, and 1.09/1000 person days from 2020 to 2022, respectively. Fifth, the confounding factors were not adjusted in Poisson regression, and only a mild reduction in restraint requirement after bundle care was performed. Further logistic regression models need to include confounding factors.

5. Conclusions

This study found increasing evidence that integrated care by translating evidence-based knowledge into clinical practice can effectively reduce PrI incidence to improve the quality of care and patients' health outcomes. The PrI care bundle for critical care patients was redesigned through multidisciplinary teamwork and organized structures with effective communication. Therefore, through integrated care through education and training, nurses can take steps to provide reliable clinical care and reduce the occurrence of PrIs.

Supplementary Materials: The following supporting information can be downloaded at: https://www.mdpi.com/article/10.3390/healthcare11152116/s1, Table S1: The cases of different sites of non-iatrogenic and iatrogenic pressure injuries.

Author Contributions: Conceptualization, R.-Y.L.; Data curation, S.-H.H.; Formal analysis, C.-A.C.; Funding acquisition, C.-G.C.; Investigation, S.-H.H., S.-F.L., W.-J.Y., S.-I.C., D.-H.C. and H.-C.L.; Methodology, W.-J.Y. and H.-C.L.; Project administration, R.-Y.L.; Resources, C.-Y.W.; Supervision, C.-A.C.; Validation, C.-Y.W., S.-F.L., S.-I.C. and D.-H.C.; Visualization, C.-Y.W. and H.-C.L.; Writing—original draft, R.-Y.L.; Writing—review and editing, C.-G.C. and C.-A.C. All authors have read and agreed to the published version of the manuscript.

Funding: This research received no external funding.

Institutional Review Board Statement: The study was conducted in accordance with the Declaration of Helsinki and approved by the Institutional Review Board of TPEVGH (TPEVGHIRB No.: 2020-07-002CC), 24 June 2020 approval.

Informed Consent Statement: Patient consent was waived because this was a retrospective study and chart review does not require informed consent.

Data Availability Statement: The datasets used in the current study are available from the corresponding author upon reasonable request.

Acknowledgments: The authors thank TYAFGH-E-112042 for supporting this study.

Conflicts of Interest: The authors declare no conflict of interest.

References

1. Padula, W.V.; Black, J.M.; Davidson, P.M.; Kang, S.Y.; Pronovost, P.J. Adverse Effects of the Medicare PSI-90Hospital Penalty System on Revenue-Neutral Hospital-Acquired Conditions. *J. Patient Saf.* **2020**, *16*, e97–e102. [CrossRef]
2. Alderden, J.; Rondinelli, J.; Pepper, G.; Cummins, M.; Whitney, J. Risk factors for pressure injuries among critical care patients: A systematic review. *Int. J. Nurs. Stud.* **2017**, *71*, 97–114. [CrossRef]
3. Chaboyer, W.P.; Thalib, L.; Harbeck, E.L.; Coyer, F.M.; Blot, S.; Bull, C.F.; Nogueira, P.C.; Lin, F.F. Incidence and Prevalence of Pressure Injuries in Adult Intensive Care Patients: A Systematic Review and Meta-Analysis. *Crit. Care Med.* **2018**, *46*, e1074–e1081. [CrossRef]
4. Lin, F.; Wu, Z.; Song, B.; Coyer, F.; Chaboyer, W. The effectiveness of multicomponent pressure injury prevention programs in adult intensive care patients: A systematic review. *Int. J. Nurs. Stud.* **2020**, *102*, 103483. [CrossRef] [PubMed]
5. Jackson, D.E.; Durrant, L.A.; Hutchinson, M.; Ballard, C.A.; Neville, S.; Usher, K. Living with multiple losses: Insights from patients living with pressure injury. *Collegian* **2018**, *25*, 409–414. [CrossRef]
6. Lovegrove, J.; Fulbrook, P.; Miles, S. Prescription of pressure injury preventative interventions following risk assessment: An exploratory, descriptive study. *Int. Wound J.* **2018**, *15*, 985–992. [CrossRef]
7. European Pressure Ulcer Advisory Panel; National Pressure Injury Advisory Panel; Pan Pacific Pressure Injury Alliance. *Prevention and Treatment of Pressure Ulcers/Injuries: Clinical Practice Guideline*, 3rd ed.; EPUAP/NPIAP/PPPIA: Westford, MA, USA, 2019.
8. Tayyib, N.; Coyer, F. Effectiveness of Pressure Ulcer Prevention Strategies for Adult Patients in Intensive Care Units: A Systematic Review. *Worldviews Evid. Based Nurs.* **2016**, *13*, 432–444. [CrossRef]
9. Anderson, M.; Finch Guthrie, P.; Kraft, W.; Reicks, P.; Skay, C.; Beal, A.L. Universal Pressure Ulcer Prevention Bundle with WOC Nurse Support. *J. Wound Ostomy Continence Nurs.* **2015**, *42*, 217–225. [CrossRef]
10. Tayyib, N.; Coyer, F. Translating Pressure Ulcer Prevention Into Intensive Care Nursing Practice: Overlaying a Care Bundle Approach with a Model for Research Implementation. *J. Nurs. Care Qual.* **2017**, *32*, 6–14. [CrossRef]
11. Santy-Tomlinson, J.; Limbert, E. Using the SSKIN care bundle to prevent pressure ulcers in the intensive care unit. *Nurs. Stand.* **2020**, *35*, 77–82.

12. Byrne, S.; Patton, D.; Avsar, P.; Strapp, H.; Budri, A.; O'Connor, T.; Nugent, L.; Moore, Z. Sub epidermal moisture measurement and targeted SSKIN bundle interventions, a winning combination for the treatment of early pressure ulcer development. *Int. Wound J.* **2022**, *20*, 1987–1999. [CrossRef]
13. Zhang, X.; Wu, Z.; Zhao, B.; Zhang, Q.; Li, Z. Implementing a Pressure Injury Care Bundle in Chinese Intensive Care Units. *Risk Manag. Healthc. Policy* **2021**, *14*, 2435–2442. [CrossRef]
14. Kennerly, S.M.; Sharkey, P.D.; Horn, S.D.; Alderden, J.; Yap, T.L. Nursing Assessment of Pressure Injury Risk with the Braden Scale Validated against Sensor-Based Measurement of Movement. *Healthcare* **2022**, *10*, 2330. [CrossRef]
15. Rivera, J.; Donohoe, E.; Deady-Rooney, M.; Douglas, M.; Samaniego, N. Implementing a Pressure Injury Prevention Bundle to Decrease Hospital-Acquired Pressure Injuries in an Adult Critical Care Unit: An Evidence-Based, Pilot Initiative. *Wound Manag. Prev.* **2020**, *66*, 20–28. [CrossRef]
16. Tayyib, N.; Asiri, M.Y.; Danic, S.; Sahi, S.L.; Lasafin, J.; Generale, L.F.; Malubay, A.; Viloria, P.; Palmere, M.G.; Parbo, A.R.; et al. The Effectiveness of the SKINCARE Bundle in Preventing Medical-Device Related Pressure Injuries in Critical Care Units: A Clinical Trial. *Adv. Skin Wound Care* **2021**, *34*, 75–80. [CrossRef]
17. Coyer, F.; Gardner, A.; Doubrovsky, A.; Cole, R.; Ryan, F.M.; Allen, C.; McNamara, G. Reducing pressure injuries in critically ill patients by using a patient skin integrity care bundle (InSPiRE). *Am. J. Crit. Care* **2015**, *24*, 199–209. [CrossRef]
18. Gupta, P.; Shiju, S.; Chacko, G.; Thomas, M.; Abas, A.; Savarimuthu, I.; Omari, E.; Al-Balushi, S.; Jessymol, P.; Mathew, S.; et al. A quality improvement programme to reduce hospital-acquired pressure injuries. *BMJ Open Qual.* **2020**, *9*, e000905. [CrossRef]
19. Lovegrove, J.; Fulbrook, P.; Miles, S. International consensus on pressure injury preventative interventions by risk level for critically ill patients: A modified Delphi study. *Int. Wound J.* **2020**, *17*, 1112–1127. [CrossRef]
20. Rêgo, A.d.S.; Furtado, G.E.; Bernardes, R.A.; Santos-Costa, P.; Dias, R.A.; Alves, F.S.; Ainla, A.; Arruda, L.M.; Moreira, I.P.; Bessa, J.; et al. Development of Smart Clothing to Prevent Pressure Injuries in Bedridden Persons and/or with Severely Impaired Mobility: 4NoPressure Research Protocol. *Healthcare* **2023**, *11*, 1361. [CrossRef]
21. Gibelli, F.; Bailo, P.; Sirignano, A.; Ricci, G. Pressure Ulcers from the Medico-Legal Perspective: A Case Report and Literature Review. *Healthcare* **2022**, *10*, 1426. [CrossRef]
22. Chao, W.-Y.; Wu, Y.-L.; Liao, W.-C. Psychometric Properties of the Taiwanese Pressure Ulcer Management Self-Efficacy Scale in Nursing Practice. *Healthcare* **2022**, *10*, 1900. [CrossRef]
23. Furtado, K.; Voorham, J.; Infante, P.; Afonso, A.; Morais, C.; Lucas, P.; Lopes, M. The Relationship between Nursing Practice Environment and Pressure Ulcer Care Quality in Portugal's Long-Term Care Units. *Healthcare* **2023**, *11*, 1751. [CrossRef]

Disclaimer/Publisher's Note: The statements, opinions and data contained in all publications are solely those of the individual author(s) and contributor(s) and not of MDPI and/or the editor(s). MDPI and/or the editor(s) disclaim responsibility for any injury to people or property resulting from any ideas, methods, instructions or products referred to in the content.

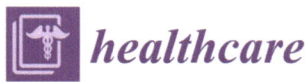

Article

Impact of Care Interventions on the Survival of Patients with Cardiac Chest Pain

Silmara Meneguin [1,*], Camila Fernandes Pollo [1], Murillo Fernando Jolo [1], Maria Marcia Pereira Sartori [2], José Fausto de Morais [3] and Cesar de Oliveira [4]

1. Department of Nursing, Botucatu Medical School, Paulista State University—Unesp, São Paulo 18618687, SP, Brazil; camilapollo@hotmail.com (C.F.P.); murilloofj@gmail.com (M.F.J.)
2. Department of Plant Production, School of Agriculture, Paulista State University—Unesp, Botucatu 18610034, SP, Brazil; maria.mp.sartori@unesp.br
3. Faculty of Mathematics, Federal University of Uberlândia, Uberlândia 38400902, MG, Brazil; jfmorais.ufu@hotmail.com
4. Department of Epidemiology & Public Health, University College London, London WC1E 6BT, UK; c.oliveira@ucl.ac.uk
* Correspondence: s.meneguin@unesp.br

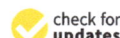

Citation: Meneguin, S.; Pollo, C.F.; Jolo, M.F.; Sartori, M.M.P.; de Morais, J.F.; de Oliveira, C. Impact of Care Interventions on the Survival of Patients with Cardiac Chest Pain. *Healthcare* 2023, *11*, 1734. https://doi.org/10.3390/healthcare11121734

Academic Editor: Christina Alexopoulou

Received: 11 May 2023
Revised: 8 June 2023
Accepted: 8 June 2023
Published: 13 June 2023

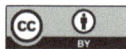

Copyright: © 2023 by the authors. Licensee MDPI, Basel, Switzerland. This article is an open access article distributed under the terms and conditions of the Creative Commons Attribution (CC BY) license (https:// creativecommons.org/licenses/by/ 4.0/).

Abstract: Background: Chest pain is considered the second most frequent complaint among patients seeking emergency services. However, there is limited information in the literature about how the care provided to patients with chest pain, when being attended to in the emergency room, influences their clinical outcomes. Aims: To assess the relationship between care interventions performed on patients with cardiac chest pain and their immediate and late clinical outcomes and to identify which care interventions were essential to survival. Methods: In this retrospective study. We analyzed 153 medical records of patients presenting with chest pain at an emergency service center, São Paulo, Brazil. Participants were divided into two groups: (G1) remained hospitalized for a maximum of 24 h and (G2) remained hospitalized for between 25 h and 30 days. Results: Most of the participants were male 99 (64.7%), with a mean age of 63.2 years. The interventions central venous catheter, non-invasive blood pressure monitoring, pulse oximetry, and monitoring peripheral perfusion were commonly associated with survival at 24 h and 30 days. Advanced cardiovascular life support and basic support life ($p = 0.0145$; OR = 8053; 95% CI = 1385–46,833), blood transfusion ($p < 0.0077$; OR = 34,367; 95% CI = 6489–182,106), central venous catheter ($p < 0.0001$; OR = 7.69; 95% CI 1853–31,905), and monitoring peripheral perfusion ($p < 0.0001$; OR = 6835; 95% CI 1349–34,634) were independently associated with survival at 30 days by Cox Regression. Conclusions: Even though there have been many technological advances over the past decades, this study demonstrated that immediate and long-term survival depended on interventions received in an emergency room for many patients.

Keywords: chest pain; assistance; critical care; emergency medical services; nursing

1. Background

Chest pain is considered the second most frequent complaint among patients seeking emergency services. On average, six million patients visit emergency centers on an annual basis due to chest pain [1]. This symptom, which can be cardiac or non-cardiac in origin, benign or life-threatening, requires prompt diagnosis and management [2].

Among cardiac diseases, acute coronary syndrome (ACS), the most common clinical symptom of coronary artery disease, is characterized by a set of manifestations of acute myocardial ischemia and is responsible for 1/5 of the causes of chest pain [3,4].

Initially, clinical manifestations of ACS occur following a decrease in local circulation due to luminal narrowing. This commonly presents as a pressure chest pain that radiates to the left or right upper limb or mandible and may be associated with cold sweating, nausea, abdominal pain, or lipothymia [5].

The published literature shows that less than 15% of ACS cases are correctly diagnosed [6]. In Canada, it is estimated that 4.6% of patients with acute myocardial infarction and 6.4% of cases with unstable angina are misdiagnosed [7]. In Brazil, the proportion of ACS patients who are diagnosed ranges from 2% to 10% [4].

Globally, heart disease has remained the leading cause of death for the last 20 years, and it represents 16% of total deaths from all causes [8]. In Brazil, besides being the main cause of death since 1960, heart disease contributes to 31% of all deaths [9,10].

These data illustrate the need for public health strategies that seek to mitigate the impact of these conditions that are the main cause of morbidity and mortality in developed and developing countries [11,12].

In the emergency room, patient care for such patients should be focused on clinical history, a survey of symptoms, research on related risk factors, physical examination, and requests for additional tests such as electrocardiogram and troponin, which should be tested every 6–12 h at least [13,14].

During this phase, nursing care is based on comprehensive care. Additionally, the nursing care plan developed in the acute stage of the disease must include the patient's basic human needs [15]. The aim of this care plan is to contribute to stabilizing the patient, reducing morbidity and mortality, and preventing further complications [11].

However, there is limited information in the literature about how the care provided to patients with chest pain, when being attended to in the emergency room, influences their clinical outcomes. Extensive research has been focused on the care provided for other conditions, such as post-cardiac arrest and HIV, among others [12,16].

Based on this gap in the literature, this investigation was carried out to answer the following questions: Is the care provided to patients with chest pain in the emergency room related to clinical outcomes? Do the interventions provided by this care have an impact on patient survival?

This study set out to verify whether the interventions performed on patients with cardiac chest pain had an impact on their immediate and late clinical outcomes as well as to identify the care interventions that could be described as survival factors.

2. Methods

This descriptive, exploratory, and retrospective study was conducted at an Emergency Center of a public institution in the State of São Paulo, from February to October 2019.

Patients of both sexes, aged 18 or older, admitted to the emergency room of the Emergency Center and hospitalized for a period of 30 days or less with chest pain due to a cardiac etiology documented in the medical record were considered eligible for the study. Patients who were hospitalized for more than 30 days were excluded.

Initially, a survey of all the daily consultations was carried out in the emergency room of the emergency center, from January to June 2018. Following this, medical records of 274 patients who presented with chest pain were retrieved; 118 were then excluded because the chest pain was attributed to a cardiac cause and 3 were excluded as they had been hospitalized for more than 30 days. Ultimately, 156 patients with cardiac chest pain were included in this analysis.

Two data collection instruments were used; the first consisted of sociodemographic and clinical data, namely date of hospital admission, data collection, date of birth, sex, origin before the admission to the emergency room, personal history, or comorbidities, diagnostic or diagnostic hypothesis, treatment (double anti-aggregation, invasive or thrombolytic interventionist), complications throughout hospitalization, and clinical outcomes (death and survival).

The second instrument documented the nursing care given towards cardiac chest pain, which was listed following the standardization proposed by the Nursing Interventions Classification (NIC). This included the following variables: heart rate (HR) and pace, neurological status, liquid balance, bladder catheterization, 12-lead electrocardiogram (ECG), peripheral venous puncture (PVP), central venous puncture (CVP), control laboratory tests, whether a chest x-ray was done, non-invasive blood pressure (NIBP), invasive blood pressure (IBP), pulse oximetry, arterial blood gases, partial oxygen pressure (PaO$_2$), oxygen therapy, peripheral perfusion, antiarrhythmic therapy, cardiac auscultation, pulmonary auscultation, 2-hourly change of position, use of anticoagulants, medications dispensed to relieve/prevent pain and ischemia, thrombolytic therapy, basic and advanced life support measures (BLS and ACLS), institution of oral nutrition, institution of enteral nutrition, transfer to intensive care unit (ICU), transfer to service hemodynamics, and use of vasoactive drug and blood transfusion [17].

To answer the study's objectives, patients were divided into two groups: Group 1 (G1) consisted of patients who were hospitalized for only 24 h, and Group 2 (G2) consisted of patients who were hospitalized for a period ranging from 25 h to 30 days. Groups 1 and 2 were not different. Their separation was done for survival measurement purposes.

Descriptive analyses were performed, initially. Pearson's chi-square test or Fisher's exact test were used to compare the interventions performed in both patient groups.

Kaplan-Meir survival curves were calculated for each type of care/intervention performed considering survival at 24 h and 30 days. The data were assessed after 30 days of follow-up with the possible outcome being discharge or death. The comparison of survival at 24 h was done using a comparison test like the Chi-square test. A Cox regression model was adjusted for survival time considering the different types of care provided using the Stepwise method to select the interventions which were more correlated to survival time.

PCA (Principal Component Analysis) was used to assess the correlation between the interventions performed and survival. The analysis used the R software version 3.6.2 and the Statistical Package for the Social Sciences (SPSS) version 20.0, Windows platform.

This research was approved by the Research Ethics Committee (protocol no. 4.011.394.).

3. Results

Based on the inclusion criteria, 153 participants were included in the study sample; of those participants, 23 were hospitalized for only 24 h (Group G1), and 130 were hospitalized for a period ranging from 25 h to 30 days (Group G2). Table 1 shows the participants' sociodemographic and clinical characteristics for G1 and G2 groups and for all participants.

Most of the participants were male 99 (64.7%), with a mean age of 63.1 years, had comorbidities (88.9%), among which high blood pressure 107 (69.9%), dyslipidemia 66 (43.1%), and diabetes 57 (37.3%) stood out as the most prevalent. Most participants had a history of smoking 83 (54.2%) and on average, received six interventions. Around one-tenth (10%) of the participants died. With the exception of the variables days of hospitalization and outcome, no statistically significant difference was identified between the statistics when comparing groups G1 and G2. In the case of the variable days of hospitalization, the result was as expected and in the case of the outcome variable, the significance was borderline.

Table 2 describes the information related to chest pain, diagnosis, and treatment for G1 and G2 groups and for all participants. The most prevalent chest pain was precordial (89.5%) associated with sweating (12.4%) and that radiated (56.9). The duration of pain for most participants (37.3%) was less than one hour and the predominant medical diagnosis was acute myocardial infarction (68.6%). Most patients were managed conservatively with the use of mainly double antiplatelet therapy (68.0%) and invasive interventional therapy (26.8%). No statistically significant association was identified between the variables and groups G1 and G2.

Table 1. Sociodemographic, clinical, and care-related characteristics of study participants. Botucatu, SP, Brazil, 2020.

Variable	G1 (n = 23)	G2 (n = 130)	Total (n = 153)	p
Sex				
Male	16 (69.6)	83 (63.8)	99 (64.7)	
Female	7 (30.4)	47 (36.2)	54 (35.3)	0.597 [1]
Age (years)				
Mean (±SD)	60.2 ± 14.2	63.6 ± 13.0	63.1 ± 13.2	0.289 [2]
Days of hospitalization				
Mean (±SD)	2.9 ± 3.6	7.7 ± 6.1	7.0 ± 6.0	<0.001
Comorbidities				
Yes	21 (91.3)	115 (88.5)	136 (88.9)	0.512 [4]
Arterial hypertension				
Yes	17 (73.9)	90 (69.2)	107 (69.9)	0.652 [1]
Dyslipidemia				
Yes	13 (56.5)	74 (56.9)	87 (56.9)	0.971 [1]
Diabetes Mellitus				
Yes	16 (69.6)	80 (63.8)	96 (62.7)	0.597 [1]
History of infarction				
Yes	3 (13.0)	21 (16.2)	24 (15.7)	0.494 [4]
Coronary artery disease				
Yes	3 (13.0)	16 (12.3)	19 (12.4)	0.572 [4]
Obesity				
Yes	2 (8.7)	10 (7.7)	12 (7.8)	0.566 [4]
History of smoking				
Yes	10 (43.5)	73 (56.2)	83 (54.2)	0.261 [1]
Smoking				
Yes	5 (21.7)	30 (23.1)	35 (22.9)	0.888 [1]
Number of interventions				
Mean (±SD)	6.3 ± 2.7	6.0 ± 2.1	6.0 ± 2.2	0.903 [3]
Outcome				
Survivals	18 (78.3)	120 (92.3)	138 (90.2)	
Deaths	5 (21.7)	10 (7.7)	15 (9.8)	0.052 [4]

[1] Pearson's chi-square test. [2] *t*-test for independent samples. [3] Mann-Whitney U test. [4] Fisher's exact test.

Table 3 describes the nursing interventions provided to the study participants. The most prevalent interventions in both groups were performing a 12-lead ECG (96.7%), monitoring pace and HR (84.3%), control laboratory tests (82.4%), and peripheral venous puncture (70.6%). On the other hand, a central venous puncture was performed more frequently in G2 than in G1 (31.0% vs. 13.3%; $p = 0.025$, respectively). Furthermore, a transfer to ICU was also more common in G2 when the groups were compared (0.00% vs. 30%; $p = 0.002$).

Table 4 displays the types of care that were associated with survival rates using the Kaplan-Meir method at 24 h and 30 days. Survival at 24 h was significantly associated with monitoring neurological status ($p < 0.0001$), central venous catheter ($p = 0.0006$), non-invasive blood pressure monitoring ($p = 0.0074$), pulse oximetry ($p = 0.0007$), and monitoring peripheral perfusion ($p \leq 0.0001$). Survival at 30 days was significantly associated with vesical catheterization ($p = 0.0093$), central venous catheter ($p \leq 0.0001$), non-invasive blood pressure monitoring ($p = 0.0019$), pulse oximetry ($p = 0.019$), peripheral perfusion monitoring ($p = 0.0006$), oxygen therapy ($p = 0.0139$), BLS/ACLS ($p < 0.0001$), use of vasoactive drug ($p = 0.0002$), and blood transfusion ($p < 0.0001$)

Table 2. Characterization of chest pain, associated symptoms, medical diagnosis, and treatment. Botucatu, 2020.

Variable	G1 (n = 23)	G2 (n = 130)	Total (n = 153)	p *
Pain site				
Precordial	20 (87.0)	119 (91.5)	137 (89.5)	
Epigastric	3 (13.0)	5 (3.8)	8 (5.2)	
Precordial and Epigastric	0 (0.0)	6 (4.6)	6 (3.9)	0.118
Pain irradiation				
Yes	15 (65.2)	72 (55.4)	87 (56.9)	0.380
Duration of pain (in hours)				
<1	14 (60.9)	43 (33.1)	57 (37.3)	
1 to 3	3 (13.0)	31 (23.8)	34 (22.2)	
4 to 23	3 (13.0)	34 (26.2)	37 (24.2)	
>24	3 (13.0)	22 (16.9)	25 (16.3)	0.084
Presence of associated symptoms				
Yes	12 (52.2)	67 (51.5)	79 (51.6)	0.955
Associated symptoms				
Sweating	4 (17.4)	15 (11.5)	19 (12.4)	
Nausea and Vomiting	1 (4.3)	10 (7.7)	11 (7.2)	
Dyspnea	0 (0.0)	10 (7.7)	10 (6.5)	
Fatigue	0 (0.0)	4 (3.1)	4 (2.6)	
Other	11 (47.8)	63 (48.5)	74 (48.4)	0.411
Medical diagnostics				
Infarction with ST-segment elevation	11 (47.8)	63 (48.50)	74 (48.3)	
Infarction without ST-segment elevation	5 (21.7)	36 (27.7)	41 (26.8)	
Unstable angina	6 (26.1)	23 (17.7)	29 (18.9)	
Stable angina	1 (4.3)	2 (1.5)	3 (2.0)	
Cardiac failure	0 (0.0)	3 (2.3)	3 (2.0)	
Angina secondary to tachyarrhythmia	0 (0.0)	3 (2.3)	3 (2.0)	0.725
Treatment				
Double anti-aggregation	19 (82.6)	85 (65.4)	104 (68.0)	
Interventional	3 (13.0)	38 (29.2)	41 (26.8)	
Thrombolytic	1 (4.3)	7 (5.4)	8 (5.2)	0.246

* Pearson Chi-square test.

Table 3. Interventions performed on study participants in the emergency room concerning groups of participants. Botucatu, SP, Brazil.

Interventions	G1 (n = 23)	G2 (n = 130)	Total (n = 153)	p
1. Monitor pace and heart rate	21 (91.3)	108 (83.1)	129 (84.3)	0.533 [1]
2. Monitor neurological state	0 (0.0)	6 (4.6)	6 (3.9)	0.592 [1]
3. Monitor liquid intake	3 (13.0)	10 (7.7)	13 (8.5)	0.416 [1]
4. Bladder catheterization	3 (13.0)	10 (7.7)	13 (8.5)	0.416 [1]
5. Performing a 12-lead ECG	22 (95.7)	126 (96.9)	148 (96.7)	0.562 [1]
6. Peripheral venous puncture	13 (56.5)	95 (73.1)	108 (70.6)	0.108 [2]
7. Central venous puncture	2 (1.5)	3 (13.0)	5 (3.3)	0.025 [1]
8. Control laboratory tests	19 (82.6)	107 (82.3)	126 (82.4)	1.000 [1]
9. Get X-ray	12 (52.2)	50 (38.5)	62 (40.5)	0.217 [2]
10. Monitor non-invasive blood pressure	7 (30.4)	26 (20.0)	33 (21.6)	0.277 [1]
11. Monitor pulse oximetry	3 (13.0)	10 (7.7)	13 (8.5)	0.416 [1]
12. Arterial blood gases	0 (0.0)	3 (2.3)	3 (2.0)	1.000 [1]
13. Administer oxygen therapy	4 (17.4)	14 (10.8)	18 (11.8)	0.479 [1]
14. Monitor peripheral perfusion	2 (8.7)	2 (1.5)	4 (2.6)	0.108 [1]
15. Use of antiarrhythmic	1 (4.3)	12 (9.2)	13 (8.5)	0.693 [1]
16. Cardiac auscultation	3 (13.0)	12 (9.2)	15 (9.8)	0.702 [1]
17. Pulmonary auscultation	3 (13.0)	19 (14.6)	22 (14.4)	1.000 [1]
18. Administer anticoagulants	11 (47.8)	50 (38.5)	61 (39.9)	0.398 [2]
19. Use of analgesics medication	1 (4.3)	11 (8.5)	12 (7.8)	0.695 [1]
20. BLS and ALS *	1 (4.3)	2 (1.5)	3 (2.0)	0.389 [1]
21. Start oral nutrition	0.00	5 (3.8)	5 (3.3)	1.000 [1]
22. Transfer to ICU	0 (0.00)	39 (30.0)	39 (25.5)	0.002 [2]
23. Transfer to hemodynamics	8 (34.8)	38 (29.2)	46 (30.1)	0.592 [2]
24. Use of vasoactive drug	5 (21.7)	25 (19.2)	30 (19.6)	0.779 [1]
25. Blood transfusion	1 (4.3)	1 (0.8)	2 (1.3)	0.279 [1]

[1] Fisher's exact test. [2] Pearson's chi-square test. * Basic Life Support and Advanced Life Support.

Table 4. Survival at 24 h and 30 days and the different types of care/interventions investigated. Botucatu, SP, Brazil.

Type of Care/Intervention	Survival Time			
	24 h	30 Days	p *	p **
1. Monitor pace and heart rate	1	0.2018	0.7222	0.6533
2. Monitor neurological state	0.966	0.1432	<0.0001	0.7051
3. Monitor liquid intake	0.9786	1.0146	0.0795	0.3138
4. Bladder catheterization	0.9786	6.7704	0.0795	0.0093
5. Performing a 12-lead ECG	1	0.3999	1	0.5271
6. Peripheral venous puncture	0.9556	0.4392	0.9766	0.5075
7. Central venous puncture	0.9797	20.4478	0.0006	<0.0001
8. Control laboratory tests	0.9259	0.7428	0.2953	0.3888
9. Get X-ray	0.967	0.9471	1	0.3305
10. Monitor non-invasive blood pressure	0.9917	9.6303	0.0074	0.0019
11. Monitor pulse oximetry	0.9857	5.5026	0.0007	0.019
12. Arterial blood gases	0.9667	0.2087	1	0.6478
13. Administer oxygen therapy	1	6.0546	1	0.0139
14. Monitor peripheral perfusion	0.9799	11.8516	<0.0001	0.0006
15. Use of antiarrhythmic	0.9797	1.2963	1	0.2549
16. Cardiac auscultation	0.971	0.6301	0.988	0.4273
17. Pulmonary auscultation	0.9695	0.0624	1	0.8027
18. Administer anticoagulants	0.9565	1.2973	0.6468	0.2547
19. Use of analgesics	0.9645	1.3717	1	0.2415
20. BLS and ALS ***	0.9733	28.7675	0.1876	<0.0001
21. Start oral nutrition	0.9662	0.5221	1	0.47
22. Transfer to ICU	0.9561	1.2891	0.419	0.2562
23. Transfer to hemodynamics	0.972	0.1492	1	0.6993
24. Use of vasoactive drug	0.9837	13.6671	0.0818	0.0002
25. Blood transfusion	0.9735	28.2419	0.0819	<0.0001

* p-value for the comparison of the survival rate at 24 h. ** 30-day survival assessment using the log-rank test. *** Basic Life Support and Advanced Life Support.

Table 5 shows the results of the Cox regression analysis. There was a statistically significant relationship between patient survival and the following interventions: central venous puncture ($p \leq 0.0001$; HR = 7.69: 95% CI 1.853–31.905), peripheral perfusion monitoring ($p \leq 0.0001$; HR = 6.835; 95% CI 1.349–34.634), BLS and ACLS (p = 0.0145; HR = 8.053; 95% CI = 1.385–46.833), and blood transfusion (p = 0.0077; HR = 34.367; 95% CI = 6.489–182.106). PCA (Principal Component Analysis).

In Figure 1 we can observe from the PCA (Principal Component Analysis) that the variables comorbidities, obesity, previous smoking, and transfer to ICU showed a negative correlation with death (i.e., no detectable/direct effect). However, the remaining variables showed a positive effect on death (i.e., red line). The survival presents a greater correlation with the interventions that are in the second quadrant of the figure (right).

Table 5. Cox regression of the types of intervention associated to a higher survival rate in 30 days. Botucatu, SP, Brazil.

Interventions	p	OR	95% CI Minimum	95% CI Maximum
Central venous puncture	<0.0001	7.69	1.853	31.905
Monitor peripheral perfusion	<0.0001	6.835	1.349	34.634
BLS and ACLS	0.0145	8.053	1.385	46.833
Blood transfusion	0.0077	34.376	6.489	182.106

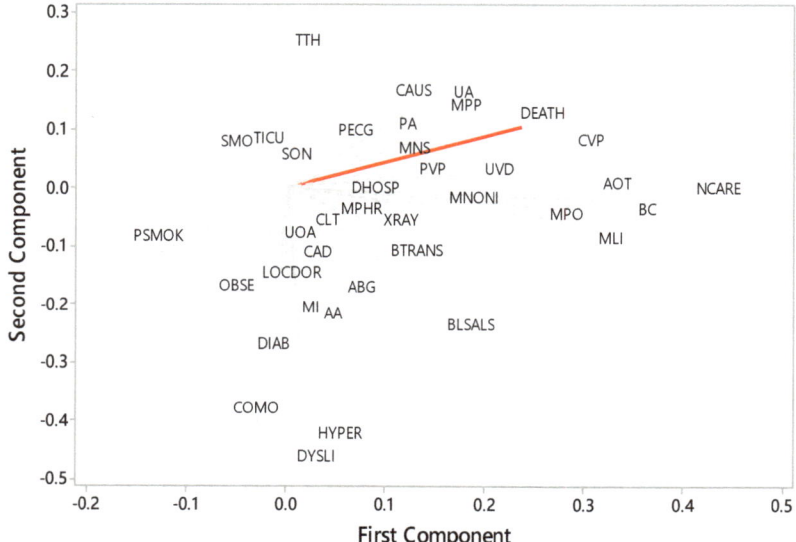

Figure 1. Principal Component Analysis (Legend: Comorbidities: COMO; Obesity: OBSE; Smoking: SMO; Previous smoking: PSMOK; Dyslipidemia: DYSLI; Diabetes: DIAB; Hypertension: HYPER; Myocardial infarction: MI; Coronary artery disease: CAD; Monitor pace and Heart Rate: MPHR; Monitor neurological state: MNS/MLI; Bladder catheterization: BC; Performing a 12-lead ECG: PECG; Peripheral venous puncture: PVP; Central venous puncture: CVP; Control laboratory tests: CLT; Getting X-ray: XRAY; Monitor non-invasive blood pressure: MNONI; Monitor pulse oximetry: MPO; Arterial blood gases: ABG; Administer oxygen therapy: AOT; Monitor peripheral perfusion: MPP; Use of antiarrhythmic: UOA; Cardiac auscultation: CAUS; Pulmonary auscultation: PA; Administer anticoagulants: AA; BLS and ALS:BLSALS; Start oral nutrition: SON; Transfer to ICU: TICU; Transfer to hemodynamics: TTH; Use of vasoactive drug: UVD; Blood transfusion: BTRANS; Number care: NCARE; Death: DEATH; Days of hospitalization: DHOSP).

4. Discussion

The nurse's role in the emergency room is crucial in determining the differential diagnosis of chest pain and the prognosis of a patient presenting with chest pain of cardiac origin which requires prompt and specific care. In this study, there was a predominance of older male participants who were hospitalized for an average of six days. This demographic is similar to that in a study conducted in another state of Brazil for patients with chest pain complaints who were admitted to the emergency room [18]. Additionally, in the literature, among patients with acute chest pain seen in the emergency room, women are less likely to have AMI or be diagnosed with ischemic heart disease [19].

With regards to comorbidities, arterial hypertension, dyslipidemia, and diabetes stood out as the most prevalent comorbidities, since they are considered classic risk factors for the onset of cardiovascular diseases. A recent study carried out among 80 patients admitted after AMI at the University Hospital of Sarajevo showed that the incidence of diabetes mellitus and obesity was significantly higher in patients aged over 45 years. Conversely, other risk factors, such as hypertension and cholesterol, were prevalent among all age groups [20].

In this study, precordial radiating pain of less than one hour's duration was the most common symptom at the time of admission. Cardiac chest pain usually lasts for a few minutes, whereas angina lasts for 2 to 10 min and AMI for more than 20 min. A sudden or continuous pain lasting several hours is rarely angina [21].

The most common diagnoses were myocardial infarction followed by unstable angina. This concurs with data from the national epidemiological profile that shows that 15% to 30% of patients with chest pain are diagnosed with acute myocardial infarction with ST-segment elevation or unstable angina [11].

Close to 10% of participants seen in the emergency room died. Studies have shown that 40–65% of deaths from AMI take place within the first hour of presentation while 80% occur within the first 24 h [22]. A high mortality rate within this timeframe could be attributed to arrhythmias such as ventricular fibrillation leading to cardiorespiratory arrest.

The ACC/AHA Joint Committee on Clinical Practice Guidelines recently developed and published a guideline for evaluation and diagnosis of chest pain. The intent of the new guideline is to outline a framework for evaluation of acute or stable chest pain syndromes or other anginal equivalents in various clinical settings, but especially in emergency departments, with emphasis on identification of ischemic and other potentially high-risk etiologies [23].

In the TIMI risk score for AMI with ST-segment elevation validation study in Porto Alegre Brazil, the mortality rate of 602 patients with a maximum age limit of 65 years was 8.6%. In the international literature, mortality rates after AMI range from 7.6 to 24% [24–26].

However, there are gender differences in the prognosis of AMI. A survey of 2042 patients revealed that in the short term (28 days), the prognosis of AMI is similar for both sexes; however, in the long term (7 years), the prognosis of male patients with AMI is worse when compared to women [27].

The most common nursing care provided was performing 12-lead ECG; however, this did not differ by patient group. It is well-established in the literature that the "door-ECG" time interval should not exceed ten minutes. Moreover, all patients with suspected ACS should have their heart pace and heart rate monitored at the initial assessment to detect cardiac arrhythmias and conduction disorders, which are frequent during the first hours of AMI. In clinical practice, it is possible that there may have been recording mistakes during this investigation due to the dynamics of care in this type of service. However, we did not evaluate for this [11].

Another frequent intervention performed by the nursing care team was to check laboratory tests. From the blood collection, it is possible to identify the biochemical markers of myocardial damage, such as troponin, CKMB, and myoglobin, which are essential for confirming a diagnosis of infarction. There is a direct association between the elevation of such biochemical markers and the risk of cardiac events; troponin is considered the most specific marker for myocardial ischemia [28].

The peripheral venous puncture for rapid drug administration, for laboratory tests, and prior to intravenous therapy was also a routine procedure in clinical practice.

After comparing the interventions performed on the two patient groups, patients in G2 were more likely to have had a central venous puncture and to be transferred to the ICU. It is possible that this care was only provided to patients who remained hospitalized, probably due to clinical complications, hemodynamic instability, and the need for vasoactive drugs.

The present study showed, after analyzing the type of patient care provided based on the length of time investigated (i.e., immediate (24 h) and delayed (30 days)), that central venous catheter, non-invasive blood pressure monitoring, pulse oximetry, and monitoring peripheral perfusion were associated with survival in both groups of patients. Patients in pain or showing signs and symptoms of respiratory failure should, therefore, receive oxygen if their oxygen saturation is below 94%. This also justifies their rigorous monitoring [11].

With regards to the wide use of pulse oximetry, it is important for nurses to have good knowledge of interpretation of its parameters to avoid any errors and, ultimately, prevent any risk to the patient [29]. In addition, nurses should understand that although pulse oximetry has a key role in the oxygen level assessment, it is not the most adequate procedure to assess a patient's ventilation capacity [30]. The pulse oximetry only measures the percentage of saturated hemoglobin with oxygen. Both the hemoglobin level and SpO_2 are needed to accurately interpret the oxygen level available for perfusion [31].

Based on the Cox regression analysis performed to answer the second specific objective of this study, monitoring peripheral perfusion and conducting peripheral venous puncture, BLS, ACLS, and blood transfusion positively contributed to increasing a patient's chance of survival at 30 days.

The use of the central venous catheter was a procedure that influenced survival positively in all analyses, corroborating the findings from clinical practice since this type of catheter is also used in the infusion of vasoactive drugs.

Our results regarding both BLS and ACLS maneuvers are in accordance with previous studies showing that adopting an immediate intervention such as cardiopulmonary resuscitation of individuals with cardiac arrest is crucial to increase their survival rate [32].

A previous study conducted with 35.065 patients who suffered cardiac arrest outside a hospital environment showed that advanced life support care was associated with survival until hospital discharge when provided initially or within six minutes from the BLS, Advanced life support care, with or without basic life support, was associated with an increased return of spontaneous circulation [33].

Limitations

There were some limitations. Incomplete documentation of patient care provided in the emergency room impacted the comprehensiveness of our analysis. Furthermore, the patient's severity score, a vital piece of information due to mortality risk prediction, was not evaluated.

Furthermore, limited information in the literature regarding the types of interventions given to patients with chest pain made it difficult to compare our results to that of published literature. Nevertheless, more research should be conducted in this area in which nursing plays a major role.

5. Conclusions

Even though there have been many technological advances over the past decades, this study demonstrated that immediate and long-term survival depended on interventions received in an emergency room for many patients.

Central venous catheter, non-invasive blood pressure monitoring, pulse oximetry and monitoring peripheral care interventions were associated to survival at 24 h and 30 days. Advanced and basic support life support, blood transfusion, central venous catheter, and monitoring peripheral perfusion influenced independently the survival rate of participants.

Author Contributions: Study design and the data collection tool: S.M. and M.F.J.; Data analysis: M.M.P.S. and J.F.d.M.; Drafting and revising of the manuscript: S.M. and C.F.P.; Approval of the final version: C.d.O. and S.M. All authors have read and agreed to the published version of the manuscript.

Funding: This work was supported by the Economic and Social Research Council (ESRC) (grant number ES/T008822/11).

Institutional Review Board Statement: The project was approved by the ethics committee of São Paulo State University (UNESP). Sao Paulo (protocol number 4.011.394).

Informed Consent Statement: Informed consent was obtained from all subjects involved in the study.

Data Availability Statement: The data that support the findings of this study are available on request from the corresponding author. The data are not publicly available due to restrictions (e.g., their containing information that compromise the privacy of research participants). All listed authors meet the authorship criteria, and all authors agree with the content of the manuscript.

Conflicts of Interest: The authors declare that this research was conducted in the absence of any commercial or financial relationships that could be construed as potential conflict of interest.

References

1. Niska, R.; Bhuiya, F.; Xu, J. National Hospital Ambulatory Medical Care Survey: 2007 emergency department summary. *Natl. Health Stat. Rep.* **2010**, *26*, 1–31.
2. Seyedhosseini-Davarani, S.; Asle-Soleimani, H.; Hossein-Nejed, H.; Jafarbaghdadi, R. Do Patients with Chest Pain Benefit from Installing Triage System in Emergency Department? *Adv. J. Emerg. Med.* **2018**, *2*, e8. [PubMed]
3. Australian Institute of Health and Welfare. *Australia's Health 2016*; Australian Institute of Health and Welfare: Canberra, Australia, 2016.
4. dos Santos, E.S.; Timerman, A. Dor Torácica na Sala de Emergência: Quem Fica e Quem Pode Ser Liberado? *Rev. Soc. Cardiol. Estado São Paulo.* **2018**, *28*, 394–402. [CrossRef]
5. Reis, A.P.P.; Ruschel, K.B.; Moraes, M.A.P.D.; Belli, K.; Saffi, M.L.; Fagundes, J.E. Risk Stratification in Chest Pain: Impact on the Diagnosis of Acute Coronary Syndrome. *Int. J. Cardiovasc. Sci.* **2020**. Available online: https://www.scielo.br/scielo.php?script=sci_arttext&pid=S2359-56472020005008203&lng=en&nrm=iso (accessed on 5 May 2023). [CrossRef]
6. Wächter, C.; Markus, B.; Schieffer, B. Cardiac causes of chest pain. *Internist* **2017**, *58*, 8–21. [CrossRef]
7. Greenslade, J.H.; Ho, A.; Hawkins, T.; Parsonage, W.; Crilly, J.; Cullen, L. Examining the translational success of an initiative to accelerate the assessment of chest pain for patients in an Australian emergency department: A pre-post study. *BMC Health Serv. Res.* **2020**, *20*, 419. [CrossRef]
8. Mahler, S.A.; Lenoir, K.M.; Wells, B.J.; Burke, G.L.; Duncan, P.W.; Case, L.D.; Herrington, D.M.; Diaz-Garelli, J.F.; Futrell, W.M.; Hiestand, B.C.; et al. Safely Identifying Emergency Department Patients With Acute Chest Pain for Early Discharge: HEART Pathway Accelerated Diagnostic Protocol. *Circulation* **2018**, *138*, 2456–2468. [CrossRef]
9. World Health Organization. WHO Reveals Leading Causes of Death and Disability Worldwide: 2000–2019. 2020. Available online: https://www.who.int/news/item/09-12-2020-who-reveals-leading-causes-of-death-and-disability-worldwide-2000-2019 (accessed on 6 July 2021).
10. Oliveira, G.M.M.; Brant, L.C.C.; Polanczyk, C.A.; Malta, D.C.; Biolo, A.; Nascimento, B.R.; Souza, M.F.M.; Lorenzo, A.R.; Fagundes Júnior, A.A.P.; Schaan, B.D.; et al. Estatística Cardiovascular—Brasil 2021. *Arq. Bras. Cardiol.* **2022**, *118*, 115–373. [CrossRef]
11. Nicolau, J.C.; Feitosa Filho, G.S.; Petriz, J.L.; Furtado, R.H.M.; Précoma, D.B.; Lemke, W.; Lopes, R.D.; Timerman, A.; Marin Neto, J.A.; Bezerra Neto, L.; et al. Brazilian Society of Cardiology Guidelines on Unstable Angina and Acute Myocardial Infarction without ST-Segment Elevation—2021. *Arq. Bras. Cardiol.* **2021**, *117*, 181–264. [CrossRef]
12. Maurício, E.C.B.; Lopes, M.C.B.T.; Batista, R.E.A.; Okuno, M.F.P.; Campanharo, C.R.V. Results of the Implementation of Integrated Care after Cardiorespiratory Arrest in a University Hospital. *Rev. Latino-Am. Enfermagem.* **2018**, *26*. Available online: https://www.scielo.br/j/rlae/a/cHg5QnYDWc6gM7xJYyN559J/?lang=pt (accessed on 6 July 2021). [CrossRef]
13. Thygesen, K.; Alpert, J.S.; Jaffe, A.S.; Chaitman, B.R.; Bax, J.J.; Morrow, D.A.; White, H.D.; Executive Group on behalf of the Joint European Society of Cardiology (ESC)/American College of Cardiology (ACC)/American Heart Association (AHA)/World Heart Federation (WHF) Task Force for the Universal Definition of Myocardial Infarction. Fourth Universal Definition of Myocardial Infarction (2018). *J. Am. Coll. Cardiol.* **2018**, *72*, 2231–2264. [CrossRef]
14. Ueng, K.C.; Chiang, C.E.; Chao, T.H.; Wu, Y.W.; Lee, W.L.; Li, Y.H.; Ting, K.H.; Su, C.H.; Lin, H.J.; Su, T.C.; et al. 2023 Guidelines of the Taiwan Society of Cardiology on the Diagnosis and Management of Chronic Coronary Syndrome. *Acta Cardiol. Sin.* **2023**, *39*, 4–96.
15. Mathias, A.L.R.; Rocha, E.F.C.; Silva, L.A.; Fedalto, C.Z.P.; da Silva, A.P. Percepção do enfermeiro frente ao paciente com suspeita de infarto agudo do miocárdio. *Rev. Recien.* **2020**, *10*. Available online: https://recien.com.br/index.php/Recien/article/view/358 (accessed on 6 July 2021).
16. Silva, A.G.; Cavalcanti, V.S.; Santos, T.S.; Bragagnollo, G.R.; Santos, K.D.; Santos, I.M.; Mousinho, K.C.; Fortuna, C.M. Integrative review of literature: Nursing care to aged people with HIV. *Rev. Bras. Enferm.* **2018**, *71* (Suppl. S2), 884–892. [CrossRef]

17. Bulechek, G.M.; Butcher, H.K.; Dochterman, J.M. Classificação das Intervenções de Enfermagem (NIC). 2010. Available online: http://site.ebrary.com/id/10894986 (accessed on 7 December 2021).
18. Pertsew, P.E.; Perozin, M.; Chaves, P.L.L. Gerenciamento do protocolo de dor torácica no setor de emergência. *Rev. Soc. Bras. Clin. Med.* **2018**, *16*. Available online: https://www.sbcm.org.br/ojs3/index.php/rsbcm/article/view/335 (accessed on 6 July 2021).
19. Miranda, A.V.D.S.; Rampellotti, L.F. Incidência da queixa de dor torácica como sintoma de infarto agudo do miocárdio em uma unidade de pronto-atendimento. *Braz. J. Pain.* **2019**, *2*. Available online: https://www.scielo.br/scielo.php?script=sci_arttext&pid=S2595-31922019000100044&lng=en&nrm=iso&tlng=en (accessed on 25 May 2023). [CrossRef]
20. Dzubur, A.; Gacic, E.; Mekic, M. Comparison of Patients with Acute Myocardial Infarction According to Age. *Med. Arch. Sarajevo. Bosnia. Herzeg.* **2019**, *73*, 23–27. [CrossRef]
21. De Filippis, A.P.; Chapman, A.R.; Mills, N.L.; De Lemos, J.A.; Arbab-Zadeh, A.; Newby, L.K.; Morrow, D.A. Assessment and Treatment of Patients with Type 2 Myocardial Infarction and Acute Nonischemic Myocardial Injury. *Circulation* **2019**, *140*, 1661–1678. [CrossRef]
22. Libby, P.; Bonow, R.; Mann, D.; Tomaselli, G.; Bhatt, D.; Solomon, S. (Eds.) *Braunwald's Heart Disease: A Textbook of Cardiovascular Medicine*, 12th ed.; Elsevier: Philadelphia, PA, USA, 2021.
23. Anderson, H.; Masri, S.C.; Abdallah, M.S.; Chang, A.M.; Cohen, M.G.; Elgendy, I.Y.; Gulati, M.; LaPoint, K.; Madan, N.; Moussa, I.D.; et al. 2022 ACC/AHA Key Data Elements and Definitions for Chest Pain and Acute Myocardial Infarction: A Report of the American Heart Association/American College of Cardiology Joint Committee on Clinical Data Standards. *Circ. Cardiovasc. Qual. Outcomes* **2022**, *15*. Available online: https://www.ahajournals.org/doi/10.1161/HCQ.0000000000000112 (accessed on 26 May 2023). [CrossRef]
24. Ersbøll, A.K.; Kjærulff, T.M.; Bihrmann, K.; Schipperijn, J.; Gislason, G.; Larsen, M.L. Geographical variation in a fatal outcome of acute myocardial infarction and association with contact to a general practitioner. *Spat. Spatio.-Temporal. Epidemiol.* **2016**, *19*, 60–69. [CrossRef]
25. Silveira, D.S.; Jaeger, C.P.; Hatschbach, L.; Manenti, E.R.F. Validação do Escore TIMI de Risco para Infarto Agudo com Supradesnivelamento do Segmento ST. *Int. J. Cardiovasc. Sci.* **2016**, *29*, 189–197.
26. Alves, L.; Polanczyk, C.A. Hospitalização por Infarto Agudo do Miocárdio: Um Registro de Base Populacional. *Arq. Bras. Cardiol.* **2020**, *115*, 916–924. [CrossRef] [PubMed]
27. Berg, J.; Björck, L.; Nielsen, S.; Lappas, G.; Rosengren, A. Sex differences in survival after myocardial infarction in Sweden. 1987–2010. *Heart* **2017**, *103*, 1625–1630. [CrossRef] [PubMed]
28. Raza, O.; Ayalew, D.; Quigg, A.; Flowers, H.; Lamont, K.; Golden, L.; Murphy, W.P. Pulse Oximetry Understanding and Application: A Survey on Nursing Staff. *J. Clin. Diagn. Res.* **2020**. Available online: https://jcdr.net/article_fulltext.asp?issn=0973-709x&year=2020&volume=14&issue=12&page=UC10&issn=0973-709x&id=14378 (accessed on 25 May 2023). [CrossRef]
29. Seeley, M.C.; McKenna, L.; Hood, K. Graduate nurses' knowledge of the functions and limitations of pulse oximetry. *J. Clin. Nurs.* **2015**, *24*, 3538–3549. [CrossRef]
30. Milutinović, D.; Repić, G.; Aranđelović, B. Clinical nurses' knowledge level on pulse oximetry: A descriptive multi-centre study. *Intensive Crit. Care Nurs.* **2016**, *37*, 19–26. [CrossRef]
31. Torp, K.D.; Modi, P.; Simon, L.V. Pulse Oximetry. In *StatPearls*; StatPearls Publishing: Treasure Island, FL, USA, 2023. Available online: http://www.ncbi.nlm.nih.gov/books/NBK470348/ (accessed on 25 May 2023).
32. Kleinman, M.E.; Brennan, E.E.; Goldberger, Z.D.; Swor, R.A.; Terry, M.; Bobrow, B.J.; Gazmuri, R.J.; Travers, A.H.; Rea, T. Part 5: Adult Basic Life Support and Cardiopulmonary Resuscitation Quality: 2015 American Heart Association Guidelines Update for Cardiopulmonary Resuscitation and Emergency Cardiovascular Care. *Circulation* **2015**, *132* (Suppl. S2), S414–S435. [CrossRef]
33. Kurz, M.C.; Schmicker, R.H.; Leroux, B.; Nichol, G.; Aufderheide, T.P.; Cheskes, S.; Grunau, B.; Jasti, J.; Kudenchuk, P.; Vilke, G.M.; et al. Advanced vs. Basic Life Support in the Treatment of Out-of-Hospital Cardiopulmonary Arrest in the Resuscitation Outcomes Consortium. *Resuscitation* **2018**, *128*, 132–137. [CrossRef]

Disclaimer/Publisher's Note: The statements, opinions and data contained in all publications are solely those of the individual author(s) and contributor(s) and not of MDPI and/or the editor(s). MDPI and/or the editor(s) disclaim responsibility for any injury to people or property resulting from any ideas, methods, instructions or products referred to in the content.

Article

Development and Validation of the CVP Score: A Cross-Sectional Study in Greece

Konstantinos Giakoumidakis [1,*], Athina Patelarou [1], Anastasia A. Chatziefstratiou [2], Michail Zografakis-Sfakianakis [1], Nikolaos V. Fotos [3] and Evridiki Patelarou [1]

1. Department of Nursing, School of Health Sciences, Hellenic Mediterranean University, 71410 Heraklion, Greece; apatelarou@hmu.gr (A.P.); mzografakis@hmu.gr (M.Z.-S.); epatelarou@hmu.gr (E.P.)
2. Cardiac Surgery Intensive Care Unit, Agia Sophia, General Pediatric Hospital of Athens, 11527 Athens, Greece; a.chatziefstratiou@yahoo.gr
3. Department of Nursing, School of Health Sciences, National & Kapodistrian University of Athens, 15771 Athens, Greece; nikfotos@nurs.uoa.gr
* Correspondence: kongiakoumidakis@hmu.gr; Tel.: +30-6973793489

Abstract: Although central venous pressure (CVP) is among the most frequent estimated hemodynamic parameters in the critically ill setting, extremely little is known on how intensive care unit (ICU) nurses use this index in their decision-making process. The purpose of the study was to develop a new questionnaire for accessing how ICU nurses use CVP measurements to address patients' hemodynamics investigating its validity and reliability. A cross-sectional study was conducted among 120 ICU nurses from four ICUs of Greece. Based on a comprehensive literature review and the evaluation by a panel of five experts, a new questionnaire, named "CVP Score", was created, having eight items. The construct validity and the reliability of the questionnaire were examined. Half of the study participants (51.7%) worked at a specialized ICU, and they had a mean [±Standard Deviation (SD)] ICU experience of 13(±7.1) years. The estimated construct validity of the newly developed tool was acceptable, while the internal consistency reliability as measured by Cronbach alpha was excellent (0.901). CVP Score had acceptable test–retest reliability ($r = 0.996$, $p < 0.001$) and split-half reliability (0.855). The CVP score is a valid and reliable instrument for measuring how critical care nurses use CVP measurements in their decision-making process.

Keywords: central venous pressure; intensive care units; questionnaire; reliability; validity

1. Introduction

Central venous pressure (CVP) is a hemodynamic parameter that has widely been monitored in the intensive care units (ICU) for assessing cardiac function, the right atrium preload, the volume status, the fluid responsiveness in critically ill patients, and it is defined as the estimated pressure in the vena cava, so can be considered as a measurement of cardiac preload and right atrial pressure [1–3]. The normal range of CVP, that is measured in a supine position via a central venous catheter placed into the subclavian or internal jugular vein, is inconsistent with different depicted values, such as 2–8 mmHg [4], 0–10 mmHg [5], or 5–15 mmHg [6], available in the currently available published research. A normal CVP waveform consists of three peak (a, c, and v waves) and two descent (x and y) phases that represent pressure changes in the right atrium. The a, c, and v waves represent atrial contraction, isovolumic ventricular contraction, and atrial systolic filling, respectively. Additionally, x descent highlights the relaxation of the atrium, while y descent highlights the early ventricular filling [5].

CVP is considered as a static indicator of cardiac preload and blood returning to the right side of the heart, despite other parameters, such as systolic pressure variation, pressure pulse variation, stroke volume variation, tidal volume challenge, respiratory change in aortic blood flow, aortic blood flow peak velocity variation, respiratory changes in pre-ejection period, variation of plethysmography, and superior–inferior vena cava collapse index, that have been recognized as dynamic indexes of fluid responsiveness [7]. Even the variability in CVP values cannot reliably predict intravenous fluid therapy responsiveness among the ICU patients' setting and the assessment of CVP values' changes remains problematic and cannot be used to determine if a patient is fluid overloaded or dehydrated [7]. At the same time, the existing evidence strongly suggests the inadequacy of single CVP measurements to guide fluid administration and resuscitation clinical decisions. It seems that only extreme measurements of CVP either low or high could guide fluid administration interventions in a more effective way [1].

Indeed, over the course of time, the usefulness and the accuracy of CVP as a strong hemodynamic and endovascular volume index has been debated and the currently available published research reveals no absolute correlation between CVP values and the total blood volume present in human circulation [8]. Osman et al. [9], in their retrospective study of 96 patients conducted in a single 24-bed medical ICU, reported that a CVP value less than 8 mmHg has a positive and negative predicted value of 51% and 65%, respectively. Additionally, Marik et al. [10] by using meta-analysis of 24 studies with a sample of 803 critically ill patient concluded that CVP is unable to predict fluid responsiveness and there is no adequate proof to support the practice of using these parameters as a guiding index of fluid administration for therapeutic purposes. In line with the above-mentioned findings, a recent single-center study of 97 critically ill patients who underwent allogeneic renal transplantation showed the superiority of stroke volume variation in guiding fluid management compared with CVP, reporting that fluid management guided by stroke volume variation monitoring, compared with CVP values evaluation, can be associated with optimal outcomes, such as the reduction in intraoperative fluid volume, the improvement of the kidney perfusion, and the promotion of postoperative recovery [11]. In favor of these data, the European Society of Intensive Care Medicine does not recommend the CVP as a measure to guide the fluids' administration and to predict the patient responsiveness to fluid therapy [8]. It seems that many inherent weaknesses of the CVP affect negatively its reliability, given that CVP values are altered by many of parameters outside the circulating blood volume, such as venous compliance, systematic vascular resistances, pulmonary hypertension, tricuspid valve insufficiency, heart failure, cardiac dysrhythmias, and conditions associated with increased intrathoracic pressure, including cardiac tamponade, tension pneumothorax, positive pressure mechanical ventilation, and positive end-expiratory pressure [12]. Additionally, CVP can be altered due to the patient body posture [13] or the presence of a valve disease [7].

Despite the inherent limitations of the CVP, that generate its sensitivity in a variety of parameters and clinical disorders, and the presence of other methods for volume status estimation and guidance to fluid administration in the clinical setting, such as transesophageal echocardiography and ultrasound-guide techniques, CVP remains the most frequent estimated hemodynamic parameter in the critically ill setting by intensivists and critical care nurses [14]. In Greece, recently the CVP measurement and estimation are among the legal professional duties of the critical care nurses [15]. It is possible that the minimal and low-cost apparatus, the easiness to be measured, and its satisfactory predictive value concerning extremely low of high values [1] are the main factors that could explain, despite the current research trends and data, its classification among the most frequently hemodynamics parameters that measured among critically ill patients in order to guide clinical decisions regarding the fluids' response and therapy.

Although many studies have been carried out in order to determine the accuracy and the reliability of CVP value for the estimation of critically ill volume and hemodynamic status [9,10,16], nothing we know regarding the extent in which critical care nurses, use CVP measurements in their decision-making process for the optimal volume, hemodynamic, and cardiovascular management of the critically ill patients, given that CVP measurements are both a frequent intervention and a legally recognized critical care nurses' professional responsibility. Attempting to add new research data to this body of knowledge was the aim of the present study in order to instigate the development of a new questionnaire for accessing how critical care nurses use CVP measurements to address patients' hemodynamics and volume status. Additionally, this study aimed to investigate the validity and reliability of this newly developed questionnaire.

2. Materials and Methods

2.1. Study Design and Participants

A cross-sectional, validation study was conducted among critical care nurses from four ICUs of two general tertiary hospitals of Greece. Being a critical care nurse was the inclusion criterion of the study. On the other hand, nurses who were unwilling to give their written consent to participate in our study and those with uncompleted filled out questionnaires were excluded. Based on these exclusion criteria, the final study sample was 120 critical care nurses. Data collection took place during a three-month period (from August to October 2018). This sample size meets the minimum requirement for the instrument validation process for at least 10 participants per questionnaire item [17].

2.2. Content Validity

Aiming to create the new questionnaire, named "CVP Score", a comprehensive literature review was conducted. In the currently available published research, we did not find any instrument which measure how nurses use CVP values in order to manage the critically ill patients and to determine their nursing care plans. At the first phase of the development of the CVP Score, 10 items have been selected for the entire questionnaire. Each item was a full sentence of specific interventions related to how nurses use CVP values in order to determine their care planning and to make clinical decisions for the critically ill patient management. Each item of the questionnaire could be answered using a 4-point Likert scale from "Never" (1 point) to "Always" (4 points).

Assessing the content validity of the new-developed questionnaire, this tool was evaluated by a five-expert panel, consisting of 2 ICU nurses, 1 intensivist, and 2 researchers with significant scientific work on intensive and critical care nursing. Each item of the questionnaire was graded by the experts as "essential", "useful but inadequate", or "unnecessary". All experts' evaluations were taken into account and finally 2 items were excluded from the questionnaire, given that their content validity ratio was lower than 0.99, according to the Lawshe Table for Minimum Values of content validity ratio [18,19]. Specifically, the content validity ratio of the first and second excluded items were 0.66 and −0.2, respectively. Subsequently, 10 people from the general population and out of our study sample provide feedback on the 8-item questionnaire, evaluating the linguistic clarity of the tool.

As presented in Tables S1 and S2, the final 8-item tool included the following questions. (1) I routinely measure CVP, two or more times during my shift; (2) I measure central venous pressure in each case of patient hemodynamic instability; (3) I estimate the fluid volume excess or deficit based on CVP values, more than the others hemodynamic parameters; (4) I plan fluid administration in low CVP values, independently of the patient blood pressure and heart rate (beats/min); (5) I plan to give diuretics and/or to limit fluid administration, independently of the patient blood pressure and heart rate (beats/min); (6) I plan my interventions (fluids administration—limitation, diuretic administration) taking into account the isolated CVP values, more than their trends—changes; (7) the inability for CVP measurement (e.g., absence of a central venous catheter, blocked lumens) negatively affects me to estimate patient hemodynamics; and (8) I predict patient fluid responsiveness by CVP values.

2.3. Data Collection

Structured face to face interviews were conducted for data collection purposes, among 120 critical care nurses from two ICUs of two general tertiary hospitals of Greece, using the "CVP Score" and a second short questionnaire on basic participants' demographics.

The CVP score ranged from 8 to 32. The high values of the CVP Score indicate high use of CVP for the nursing assessment of patients' hemodynamic and volume status, while low values are indicative that nurses considered CVP as a poor clinical tool in order to estimate patients' hemodynamics and to plan their provided care based on its values. An optimal cut-off point could be the median value of CVP Score and in our previous manuscript [20] we had defined the value of 16 as the value that marks the high (>16) and low (≤16) values of the CVP Score. At the second stage (second assessment), the participants re-answer the questionnaire through phone interviews, after one month from the first assessment, using the same order, to avoid memory effect on test and retest measurements.

Furthermore, data gathering purposes were served through a short questionnaire on basic participants' demographic characteristics, such as age, gender, educational level (undergraduate and postgraduate), experience as clinical nurse, experience in the ICU setting and ICU type (general or specialized)

2.4. Ethics

Written permission was given from the ethics committee of both of the hospitals (234/18-07-2018 and 36382/31-07-2018). Precautions took place to protect the privacy and anonymity of the participant subjects and the confidentially of their data and information, while participants gave their sign informed consent. The collected data were used only for the purpose of the present study. All the stages of the research were carried out in full accordance with the ethical standards of the Helsinki Declaration of 1975, as revised in 2013.

2.5. Statistical Analysis

Quantitative and qualitative variables were expressed as mean [±Standard Deviation (SD)] values and absolute–relative frequencies, respectively. Construct validity was described by calculating the Pearson's correlation coefficient r of the scores of the participants' responses to an item with their total scores. The Cronbach alpha coefficient was calculated for the internal consistency reliability of the entire questionnaire. Pearson's rank correlation coefficient was performed to measure the level of agreement between responses at test and re-test, while the Spearman–Brown formula was used for computing the split-half reliability. The IBM SPSS 24.0 for Window software (Armonk, NY, USA: IBM Corp) was used for our statistical analysis purposes.

3. Results

3.1. Demographics and Descriptive Statistics

As shown in Table 1, the mean (±SD) age of our study participants was 42.3 ± 6.1 years, while the majority of our sample was female subjects (71.7%), graduates of technological tertiary education (88.3%), and had no postgraduate education (66.7%). In addition, half of the study participants' (51.7%) worked at a specialized ICU, and their mean (±SD) clinical and ICU experience was 17.3 (±6.8) and 13(±7.1) years, respectively (Table 1). Finally, the mean (±SD) and the median (Interquartile range) CVP Score were 15.8 (±5.7) and 16 (10.7), respectively.

3.2. Association between Variables

In a previous manuscript, we have shown the correlation between independent variables, such as gender, educational level (basic and postgraduate), ICU type, clinical experience, and experience in an ICU setting, and only the male gender was found as a significant predictor of increased CVP Score values that indicate the higher use of CVP by critical care nurses [20].

3.3. Construct Validity

As aforementioned and summarized in Table 2, construct validity was evaluated with the Pearson's correlation coefficient r of the scores of participants' responses to an item with their total scores. All the calculated values were statistically significant and each obtained Person Correlation coefficient value was greater than the critical value from the Pearson's Correlation Table at 118 (N-2) degrees of freedom.

Table 1. Demographic characteristics of study participants.

	Mean (±SD)
Age (years)	42.3 (6.1)
Clinical experience (years)	17.3 (6.8)
ICU experience (years)	13 (7.1)
	n (%)
Gender	
Males	34 (28.3)
Females	86 (71.7)
Basic educational level	
University tertiary	14 (11.7)
Technological tertiary	106 (88.3)
Postgraduate education	
Yes	40 (33.3)
No	80 (66.7)
ICU type	
General	58 (48.3)
Specialized	62 (51.7)

ICU: Intensive care unit, SD: Standard deviation.

Table 2. Correlation of each item score with their total scores.

		Q1	Q2	Q3	Q4	Q5	Q6	Q7	Q8	Total
Q1	Pearson Correlation	1	0.745	0.522	0.326	0.461	0.420	0.396	0.422	0.731
	p-value		<0.001	<0.001	<0.001	<0.001	<0.001	<0.001	<0.001	<0.001
Q2	Pearson Correlation	0.745	1	0.627	0.413	0.509	0.358	0.489	0.536	0.791
	p-value	<0.001		<0.001	<0.001	<0.001	<0.001	<0.001	<0.001	<0.001
Q3	Pearson Correlation	0.522	0.627	1	0.772	0.657	0.585	0.477	0.571	0.841
	p-value	<0.001	<0.001		<0.001	<0.001	<0.001	<0.001	<0.001	<0.001
Q4	Pearson Correlation	0.326	0.413	0.772	1	0.732	0.652	0.326	0.578	0.757
	p-value	<0.001	<0.001	<0.001		<0.001	<0.001	<0.001	<0.001	<0.001
Q5	Pearson Correlation	0.461	0.509	0.657	0.732	1	0.627	0.267	0.509	0.760
	p-value	<0.001	<0.001	<0.001	<0.001		<0.001	0.003	<0.001	<0.001
Q6	Pearson Correlation	0.420	0.358	0.585	0.652	0.627	1	0.562	0.680	0.771
	p-value	<0.001	<0.001	<0.001	<0.001	<0.001		<0.001	<0.001	<0.001
Q7	Pearson Correlation	0.396	0.489	0.477	0.326	0.267	0.562	1	0.668	0.681
	p-value	<0.001	<0.001	<0.001	<0.001	0.003	<0.001		<0.001	<0.001

Table 2. *Cont.*

		Q1	Q2	Q3	Q4	Q5	Q6	Q7	Q8	Total
Q8	Pearson Correlation	0.422	0.536	0.571	0.578	0.509	0.680	0.668	1	0.803
	p-value	<0.001	<0.001	<0.001	<0.001	<0.001	<0.001	<0.001		<0.001
Total	Pearson Correlation	0.731	0.791	0.841	0.757	0.760	0.771	0.681	0.803	1
	p-value	<0.001	<0.001	<0.001	<0.001	<0.001	<0.001	<0.001	<0.001	

Furthermore, a factor analysis was performed. Specifically, the KMO measure of sampling adequacy was 0.806 and Bartlett's test of sphericity was 648.380, df = 28, $p < 0.001$. Factor analysis indicated that there are two principal factors in the model, and these accounted for 72.24%, as presented in Table 3. The first factor (F1) includes item 1 (I routinely measure CVP, two or more times during my shift) and its contribution was 59.326%. The second factor (F2) consists of item 2 (I measure central venous pressure in each case of patient hemodynamic instability) and the variance explained by this factor was 12.920% (Table 3). Cronbach's alpha was 0.702 and 0.251 for F1 and F2, respectively.

Table 3. Exploratory factors and explained variance after rotation for the CVP score.

Item	Initial Eigenvalues			Extraction Sums of Squared Loadings			Rotation Sums of Squared Loadings [a]
	Total	% of Variance	Cumulative %	Total	% of Variance	Cumulative %	Total
Q1	4.746	59.326	59.326	4.746	59.326	59.326	4.191
Q2	1.034	12.920	72.246	1.034	12.920	72.246	3.624
Q3	0.904	11.306	83.552				
Q4	0.436	5.453	89.005				
Q5	0.320	4.004	93.010				
Q6	0.256	3.194	96.203				
Q7	0.158	1.977	98.181				
Q8	0.146	1.819	100.000				

Extraction Method: Principal Component Analysis. [a] When components are correlated, sums of squared loadings cannot be added to obtain a total variance.

3.4. Instrument Internal Consistency Reliability

The Cronbach alpha was 0.901 for the entire questionnaire.

3.5. Test–Retest Reliability

By using test–retest reliability coefficient correlation analysis, a high positive correlation was observed between the total scores of the two applications ($r = 0.996$, $p < 0.001$). The measurements of the CVP Score are depicted via a scatter plot in Figure 1. More analytically, 100 participants had the same score on both assessments (test and retest) and 20 gave different scores. From those who had different scores and answers the majority (14 participants) had higher, by one point, CVP Score between the two assessments. The remaining six critical care nurses had a two-point difference between the two measurements.

3.6. Split-Half Reliability

The split-half reliability was computed to be 0.855 using the Spearman–Brown formula.

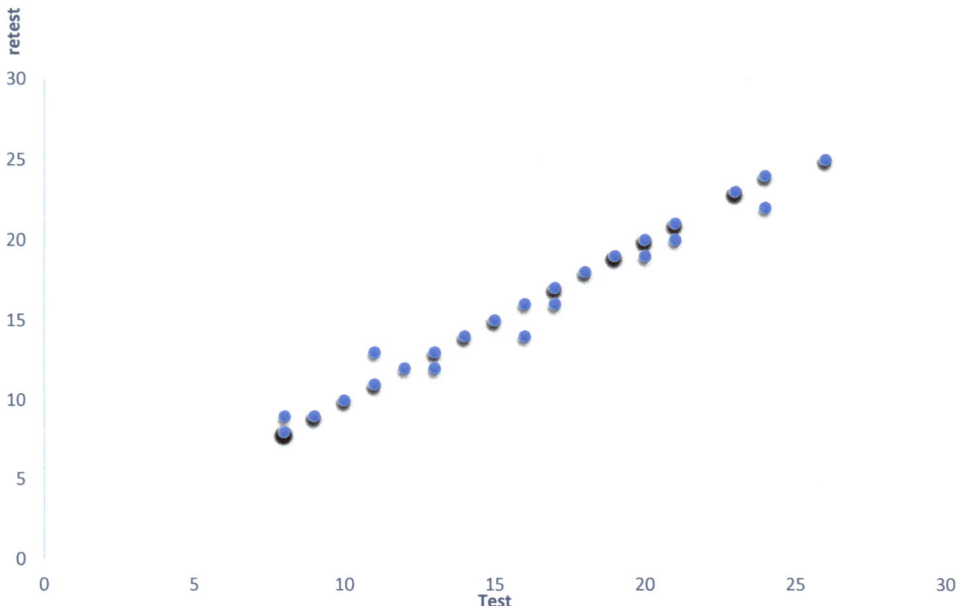

Figure 1. Scatter plot of the CVP Score test–retest measurements.

4. Discussion

According to the main aim of the present study, we developed a new instrument in order to measure how ICU nurses use CVP in order to guide their planning, clinical decisions, interventions, and fluid administration titration for the optimal management of the critically ill patient. To the best of our knowledge, this new-developed tool named "CVP Score" was the first instrument for the above-mentioned purpose, and this tool is unique in the current literature. Another important aim of the present study was to test the validity and reliability of this newly developed instrument. According to the findings of our study, "CVP Score" is a valid and reliable instrument that intends to provide researchers a significant and acceptable tool for assessing the extent of CVP values use by critical care clinicians for ICU patients in the planning of care and decision-making.

The knowledge on how critical care nurses use CVP measurements for their care planning is of utmost importance because there is not much information on this subject. Although, it is evident that CVP is the most frequent hemodynamic parameters that are estimated in the ICU environment; at the same time, we have a full absence of unambiguous proof regarding the way of CVP values incorporation in the daily nursing clinical practice. Theoretically, a significant probability is that critical care nurses estimate CVP values but they do not use these measurements to guide their clinical decisions, based on the current available literature results. Then, again, another probability is that CVP measurements operate, in critical care nurses' considerations and thoughts, as predictors of patients' hemodynamics and guide for their fluid therapy. The existence of a questionnaire, such as the "CVP Score", could provide a tool for both replying to the above questions and addressing the vision of critical care nurse on the value of CVP.

At the same time, future research projects findings with the use of the CVP score could be used productively. The mapping of the critical care nurses' considerations of CVP values during their clinical decision-making is the first step for their educational needs' evaluation in the context of continuing professional education. For instance, the finding that critical care nurses base, to a considerable degree, their clinical decisions on the estimated CVP values to manage the hemodynamic and volume status of ICU patients could work as an alarming sign and alongside a motivation to establish educational interventions on evidence-based nursing in the clinical setting aiming to provide documented, improved, and updated research evidence on this topic. Likewise, the research community could investigate whether CVP measurements are used and interpreted with different point of views in different ICU settings, such as general ICU or specialized ICU (cardiac surgery, neurosurgical ICU). Based on our professional experience, we can state the tendency of critical care nurses to overestimate CVP values in specialized cardiovascular ICUs, such as cardiac and cardiac surgery ICUs, but, that being said, nurses who provide intensive nursing care to patients in general ICUs often underestimate the value of CVP measurements, considering CVP as not a helpful parameter that cannot be taking into account in their clinical decision-making process regarding the prediction of the hemodynamic and overall patients' fluid balance.

Validity is defined as the extent to which an instrument measures exactly what it is supposed to measure without mistaking it with another issue, while reliability is the extent to which an instrument gives consistent results in repeated measurements under similar conditions [17]. Assessing the validity of the "CVP Score", it followed that there needed to be the appropriate methodology to ensure its content validity during the development of our instrument. Additionally, the evaluated construct validity of the "CVP Score", through the correlation of each item score with the total score, emerged as acceptable [18]. Likewise, construct validity assessed by factor analysis, based on our findings of KMO and Bartlett's tests that indicated that our sample was excellently adequate and the correlation between the data was sufficient for factor analysis, respectively [18]. The validity of our 8-item instrument was found to be 72.24%, demonstrating that CVP Score can achieve the purpose it wants to measure [18]. The main contributive factor was the item I (I routinely measure CVP, two or more times during my shift) explained the 59.326% of the total variance, while the second item (I measure central venous pressure in each case of patient hemodynamic instability) explained the remaining 12.920%.

On the other hand, assessing the reliability of our new-developed questionnaire we observed that "CVP Score" had an excellent Cronbach alpha coefficient, given that this parameter should have values higher than 0.59 and lower than 0.95 [18]. In addition, test–retest reliability was computed as acceptable and, finally, aiming to estimate the split-half reliability of our tool we found a strong positive correlation, which highlights our questionnaire acceptability [18].

Despite the significance of the present study, the main limitation was the full absence of a valid and reliable instrument which investigates the same issue. Thereafter, the examination of parameters that evaluate how accurately the tool measures the outcome it was designed to measure, the association of the tool with accepted standards, and its ability to predict future test results, such as the criterion, concurrent, and predictive validity of the "CVP Score", respectively, were inapplicable [18,21].

5. Conclusions

All things considered, and according to the validity and reliability analysis of our new-developed questionnaire, this tool is a valid and reliable instrument that could be used in the critical care setting, aiming to measure the extent to which critical care nurses use CVP measurements in their clinical decision-making process for the optimal volume, hemodynamic, cardiovascular monitoring, and management of the critically ill patients. It seems that ICU clinicians and researchers could use "CVP Score" to add new data to the above-mentioned limited body of knowledge. Our study significance could be underlying by the originality of the evaluated tool, taking into account that it is the first one to serve the above-mentioned research purpose. Although, based on the current literature, the value of the CVP measurement as a reliable index of cardiovascular and intravascular blood volume status, which can guide the fluid administration therapy and predict fluid responsiveness is controversial, the measurement of CVP remains a standard professional skill and responsibility of ICU clinicians, including critical care nurses. Our study limitations show that further research is needed, using the "CVP Score" on greater samples and in different ICU settings, countries, and healthcare systems.

Supplementary Materials: The following supporting information can be downloaded at: https://www.mdpi.com/article/10.3390/healthcare11111543/s1, Table S1: CVP Score (in Greek); Table S2: CVP Score (in English).

Author Contributions: Conceptualization, K.G.; methodology, K.G. and A.P.; software, K.G. and M.Z.-S.; validation, K.G. and A.A.C.; formal analysis, K.G.; investigation, K.G., A.P., N.V.F. and M.Z.-S.; data curation, E.P., A.P. and N.V.F; writing—original draft preparation, K.G.; writing—review and editing, K.G. and A.A.C.; supervision, K.G. and E.P.; project administration, K.G. All authors have read and agreed to the published version of the manuscript.

Funding: This research received no external funding.

Institutional Review Board Statement: The study was conducted in accordance with the Declaration of Helsinki, and approved by the Institutional Review Board (or Ethics Committee) of General Hospital of Athens "Evaggelismos" (234/18-07-2018) and University Hospital of Larisa (36382/31-07-2018).

Informed Consent Statement: Informed consent was obtained from all subjects involved in the study. Written informed consent has been obtained from the patients to publish this paper.

Data Availability Statement: The data presented in this study are available on request from the corresponding author.

Conflicts of Interest: The authors declare no conflict of interest.

References

1. De Backer, D.; Vincent, J.L. Should we measure the central venous pressure to guide fluid management? Ten answers to 10 questions. *Crit. Care* **2018**, *22*, 43. [CrossRef] [PubMed]
2. Guarnieri, M.; Belleti, A.; Saglietti, F.; Bignami, E. Central venous pressure as a predictor of fluid responsiveness. Is this all you need? *Gen. Med.* **2016**, *4*, 1000228. [CrossRef]
3. Sondergaard, S.; Parkin, G.; Aneman, A. Central venous pressure: Soon an outcome-associated matter. *Curr. Opin. Anaesthesiol.* **2016**, *29*, 179–185. [CrossRef] [PubMed]
4. Broch, O.; Hummitzsch, L.; Renner, J.; Meybohm, P.; Albrecht, M.; Rosenthal, P.; Rosenthal, A.C.; Steinfath, M.; Bein, B.; Gruenewald, M. Feasibility and beneficial effects of an early goal directed therapy after cardiac arrest: Evaluation by conductance method. *Sci. Rep.* **2021**, *11*, 5326. [CrossRef] [PubMed]
5. Bootsma, I.T.; Boerma, E.C.; de Lange, F.; Scheeren, T.W.L. The contemporary pulmonary artery catheter. Part 1: Placement and waveform analysis. *J. Clin. Monit. Comput.* **2022**, *36*, 5–15. [CrossRef] [PubMed]
6. Oh, C.; Noh, C.; Hong, B.; Shin, S.; Jeong, K.; Lim, C.; Kim, Y.H.; Lee, S.; Lee, S.Y. Is measurement of central venous pressure required to estimate systemic vascular resistance? A retrospective cohort study. *BMC Anesthesiol.* **2021**, *21*, 310. [CrossRef] [PubMed]
7. Alvarado Sánchez, J.I.; Amaya Zúñiga, W.F.; Monge García, M.I. Predictors to Intravenous Fluid Responsiveness. *J. Intensive Care Med.* **2018**, *33*, 227–240. [CrossRef] [PubMed]
8. Cecconi, M.; Aya, H.D. Central venous pressure cannot predict fluid-responsiveness. *Evid. Based Med.* **2014**, *19*, 63. [CrossRef] [PubMed]
9. Osman, D.; Ridel, C.; Ray, P.; Monnet, X.; Anguel, N.; Richard, C.; Teboul, J.L. Cardiac filling pressures are not appropriate to predict hemodynamic response to volume challenge. *Crit. Care Med.* **2007**, *35*, 64–68. [CrossRef] [PubMed]
10. Marik, P.E.; Baram, M.; Vahid, B. Does central venous pressure predict fluid responsiveness? A systematic review of the literature and the tale of seven mares. *Chest* **2008**, *134*, 172–178. [CrossRef] [PubMed]
11. Zhang, Y.; Chen, H.; Yu, W.; Jiang, H.; Zhan, C. Effectiveness of central venous pressure versus stroke volume variation in guiding fluid management in renal transplantation. *Am. J. Transl. Res.* **2021**, *13*, 7848–7856. [PubMed]
12. Cecconi, M.; De Backer, D.; Antonelli, M.; Beale, R.; Bakker, J.; Hofer, C.; Jaeschke, R.; Mebazaa, A.; Pinsky, M.R.; Teboul, J.L.; et al. Consensus on circulatory shock and hemodynamic monitoring. Task force of the European Society of Intensive Care Medicine. *Intensive Care Med.* **2014**, *40*, 1795–1815. [CrossRef] [PubMed]
13. Ukere, A.; Meisner, S.; Greiwe, G.; Opitz, B.; Benten, D.; Nashan, B.; Fischer, L.; Trepte, C.J.C.; Reuter, D.A.; Haas, S.A.; et al. The influence of PEEP and positioning on central venous pressure and venous hepatic hemodynamics in patients undergoing liver resection. *J. Clin. Monit. Comput.* **2017**, *31*, 1221–1228. [CrossRef] [PubMed]

14. Roger, C.; Muller, L.; Riou, B.; Molinari, N.; Louart, B.; Kerbrat, H.; Teboul, J.L.; Lefrant, J.Y. Comparison of different techniques of central venous pressure measurement in mechanically ventilated critically ill patients. *Br. J. Anaesth.* **2017**, *118*, 223–231. [CrossRef] [PubMed]
15. Official Government Gazette of the Hellenic Republic, Second Issue. Responsibilities and Duties of the National Healthcare System and the Public Primary Healthcare System Registered Nurses. 2022. Available online: https://sepdype.gr/kathikondologio-nosileytvn-fek-4262-10-8-22/ (accessed on 22 February 2023).
16. Dellinger, R.P.; Levy, M.M.; Rhodes, A.; Annane, D.; Gerlach, H.; Opal, S.M.; Sevransky, J.E.; Sprung, C.L.; Douglas, I.S.; Jaeschke, R.; et al. Surviving Sepsis Campaign Guidelines Committee including the Pediatric Subgroup. Surviving Sepsis Campaign: International guidelines for management of severe sepsis and septic shock. *Intensive Care Med.* **2013**, *39*, 165–228. [CrossRef] [PubMed]
17. Kimberlin, C.L.; Winterstein, A.G. Validity and reliability of measurement instruments used in research. *Am. J. Health Syst. Pharm.* **2008**, *65*, 2276–2284. [CrossRef] [PubMed]
18. Galanis, P. *Research Methodology in Health Sciences*, 1st ed.; Kritiki Editions: Athens, Greece, 2017; pp. 221–272.
19. Zeraati, M.; Alavi, N.M. Designing and validity evaluation of Quality of Nursing Care Scale in Intensive Care Units. *J. Nurs. Meas.* **2014**, *22*, 461–471. [CrossRef] [PubMed]
20. Giakoumidakis, K.; Fotos, N.V.; Chatziefstratiou, A.A.; Dokoutsidou, E.; Brokalaki, H. The use of central venous pressure for the assessment of patients' hemodynamics. *Eur. J. Pharmaceut. Med. Res.* **2019**, *6*, 646–650.
21. Chobanian, A.V.; Bakris, G.L.; Black, H.R.; Cushman, W.C.; Green, L.A.; Izzo, J.L., Jr.; Jones, D.W.; Materson, B.J.; Oparil, S.; Wright, J.T., Jr.; et al. Seventh report of the joint national committee on prevention, detection, evaluation, and treatment of high blood pressure. *Hypertension* **2003**, *42*, 1206–1252. [CrossRef] [PubMed]

Disclaimer/Publisher's Note: The statements, opinions and data contained in all publications are solely those of the individual author(s) and contributor(s) and not of MDPI and/or the editor(s). MDPI and/or the editor(s) disclaim responsibility for any injury to people or property resulting from any ideas, methods, instructions or products referred to in the content.

Article
Quality of Life and Family Support in Critically Ill Patients following ICU Discharge

Konstantina Avgeri, Epaminondas Zakynthinos, Vasiliki Tsolaki, Markos Sgantzos, George Fotakopoulos and Demosthenes Makris *

Department of Medical School, University of Thessaly, 41110 Larissa, Greece
* Correspondence: appollon7@hotmail.com; Tel.: +30-6943706079

Abstract: Background: Following discharge from the intensive care unit (ICU), critically ill patients may present cognitive dysfunction and physical disability. Objectives: To investigate the quality of life (QoL) of patients following discharge from ICU, physical performance and lung function and to assess the role of support by family members and friends. Methods: This prospective study was conducted in the University Hospital of Larissa Greece between 2020 and 2021. Patients hospitalized at the ICU for at least 48 h were included and assessed at hospital discharge, at 3 and at 12 months later. The research implements of the study were a dedicated questionnaire and the SF-36 health questionnaire for the appraisal of the QoL. Lung function changes were assessed by spirometry and physical performance by the 6-min walking test (6MWT). Results: One hundred and forty-three participants were included in the study. The mean (SD) of the physical and mental health SF-36 scores at hospital discharge, 3 and 12 months were 27.32 (19.59), 40.97 (26.34) and 50.78 (28.26) ($p < 0.0001$) and 42.93 (17.00), 55.19 (23.04) and 62.24 (23.66), ($p < 0.0001$), respectively. The forced expiratory volume in one second and 6MWT significantly improved over 12 months. Patients who were supported by two or more family members or patients who were visited by their friends >3 times/week presented better scores in the physical and mental SF36 domains at 12 months. Conclusion: This study shows that the quality of life of Greek patients who were discharged from the ICU can be positively affected both by the support they receive from their family environment and friends.

Keywords: ICU; patients' support; family support; PICS; quality of life; critical care

1. Introduction

Intensive care unit (ICU) hospitalization is a considerably stressful situation both for patients and their families [1,2] and has various physical and mental implications. Patients following ICU management may present reduced lung function [3], neuromuscular dysfunction, anxiety and depression. Six months following ICU discharge, patients showed reduced functional and pulmonary capacity, while an improvement was observed at 12 months after discharge [3]. These disorders in physical, intellectual and mental health have been described as post-ICU traumatic syndrome [1] and may be present for years, compromising the QoL of patients [4,5]. Family members may have an important role in the management of a critical illness, because they are often responsible for making decisions that the patients are unable to make on their own. Studies show that more than 50% of patients have to be taken care of by family members [6,7]. In this respect, family members' support is pivotal in improving the patients' health by contributing to quality care [8]. In turn, this has an impact on the lives of those family members. Indeed, when a patient is at the ICU in critical condition, family members may also suffer from symptoms such as anxiety, acute stress disorder, post-traumatic stress disorder, depression and complicated grief [9]. In this respect, the long-term impact of a critical disease on the QoL of both patients and family and the role of family in supporting critical care patients are important for planning effective supportive healthcare networks. Nevertheless, data regarding the impact of family support on ICU patients' post-ICU, especially in Greece, are limited.

In this study we aimed to investigate the QoL of ICU patients after their discharge from a Greek ICU and to evaluate the impact of family on their QoL over a one-year period. Furthermore, we aimed to assess lung functional changes and physical performance over this period.

2. Methods

This was a prospective study conducted in a tertiary hospital in Larissa, Greece, between 2020 and 2021. Patients were included if they (a) were discharged from the ICU following >48 h hospitalization and (b) were able to perform spirometry and the six-minute walking test (6MWT) at hospital discharge based on treating physicians' decisions and agreed to complete a questionnaire assessing the QoL and support received in daily activities.

The study was approved by the local ethics committee of the University Hospital of Larissa (No. 43704). Informed consent was obtained by the patient or next of kin.

2.1. Study Outcomes

The relationship between the overall SF-36 score at 12 months following hospital discharge and the support in daily activities (hours/day) received by family members and friends in total was the primary outcome in the study. Secondarily, we assessed the exercise performance by the 6MWT and lung function by spirometry.

2.2. Data Collection

Participants were evaluated at hospital discharge at 3 and 12 months. Patient medical records were evaluated to obtain demographic data, the severity of critical illness by the Acute Physiology and Chronic Health Evaluation (APACHE II) score, cause of admission, length of ICU stay, medical problems, medications and QoL variables.

The criteria for ICU admission/discharge or hospital discharge were left to the discretion of the treating physicians.

2.3. Questionnaire Interview

A dedicated questionnaire and an SF-36 questionnaire were implemented to assess the role of family support and the QoL. The questionnaire included items assessing the support received by spouses, family and friends based on the previous literature [6,10]. Data were adjusted for segregated care hours. Specifically, support received by spouses/family was classified as 1–4 h daily, 4–8 h daily and 24 h daily. Support received by friends was classified arbitrarily as every day, 3–4 times/week, once/week, 1–2 times/month and never. The SF-36 questionnaire includes multi-item scales measuring each of eight generic health concepts: physical functioning (PF), role limitations due to physical health problems (RP), bodily pain (BP), general health perceptions (GH), vitality (VT) tapping energy levels and fatigue, social functioning (SF), role limitations due to emotional problems (RE) and mental health (MH). Each item is weighted with an additive scaling to calculate the final domain score. A high score indicates a low impairment, and a low score designates an important impairment. The questionnaire is valid for the Greek population. In the present study, we arbitrarily used the median scores of participants in the physical and mental components of the questionnaire to classify patients as those with improved scores ($\geq$ median) and those with deteriorating scores (< median). Completion of the questionnaires was not during the scheduled interviews. The schedule was carried out by telephone communication. The questionnaires were completed in person by participants in outpatient clinics. In cases where the presence of the participant in the hospital was not possible, the evaluation was performed at home. In cases where the participant was not able to complete the questionnaire alone, the questions were answered with the assistance of the next of kin.

2.4. Respiratory Function Assessment

Lung function tests included spirometry to assess the forced expiratory volume in one second, (FEV1) and forced vital capacity of the lungs (FVC). Spirometry was performed at baseline and at the end of each time period with a computerized system. This system, which meets the ATS standards, was calibrated every day with standardized techniques according to the guidelines [11]. Pulse oximetric saturation (SpO2) was recorded immediately before each measurement using pulse oximetry (Nonin 8500 M; Nonin Medical; Minneapolis, MN, USA).

2.5. 6-Min Walk (6MWT)

The 6MWT was performed indoors about the same time of day along a 100-foot flat, straight, enclosed hallway with a hard surface that was seldom traveled. The walking course was 30 m in length, and it was marked every 3 m. Instructions to patients were given according to the accepted recommendations. The patient should sit at rest in a chair located near the starting position for at least 10 min before the test started. Clothing and shoes should be appropriate for walking. During that time, oxygen saturation, pulse and blood pressure were measured and baseline dyspnea was assessed using the Borg scale. A physician should stand near the starting line during the test without walking with the patient. Only the standardized phrases for encouragement were used during the test. When the test was finished, the post-walk Borg dyspnea, oxygen saturation and pulse rate were recorded, as well as the total distance covered [12].

2.6. Statistical Analysis

Data are expressed as mean (standard deviation (SD)) or median ((interquartile range (IQR)) or n (%). Normality was assessed by the Shapiro–Wilcoxon test. Comparisons between patients were performed using a Mann–Whitney test for continuous variables by *t*-test and nonparametric test. The means of two or more independent groups were compared by one-way ANOVA. All statistical tests were 2-sided. A result was considered statistically significant when $p < 0.05$. Analyses were performed using the SPSS v.25 software (ILLINOIS, USA).

3. Results

Overall, 143 patients were included in the study (Figure 1). Sociodemographic characteristics and baseline clinical characteristics of participants are shown in Tables 1 and 2, respectively.

Table 1. Social and demographic characteristics of participants.

Age, years		56.8 (17.49)
Female Sex, n (%)		57 (39.86)
	Family Status	
Married, n (%)		106 (74.12)
Not-married, n (%)		31 (21.68)
Widow/er, n (%)		6 (4.20)
	Accommodation	
Urban, n (%)		76 (56.70)
Daily area, n (%)		34 (25.40)
Agricultural, n (%)		24 (17.90)
	Education	
Basic education, n (%)		28 (19.59)
High School graduates, n (%)		86 (60.15)
Technical School graduates, n (%)		6 (4.19)
University graduates, n (%)		10 (6.99)
Post graduate training, n (%)		3 (2.09)
No education, n (%)		10 (6.99)

Table 1. Cont.

Type of Profession	
State employee, n (%)	13 (9.09)
Private employee, n (%)	25 (17.5)
Freelance, n (%)	9 (6.30)
Farmer, n (%)	10 (6.9)
Worker, n (%)	6 (4.19)
Housekeeper, n (%)	14 (9.80)
Retired, n (%)	52 (36.36)
University student, n (%)	5 (3.49)
Unemployed, n (%)	9 (6.29)
Rehabilitation after ICU, n (%)	70 (48.9)
Time to return to daily routine after ICU	
1–6 months, n (%)	58 (40.5)
6–12 months, n (%)	31 (21.7)
>12 months, n (%)	54 (37.3)

Data are presented as the mean (SD) unless otherwise indicated.

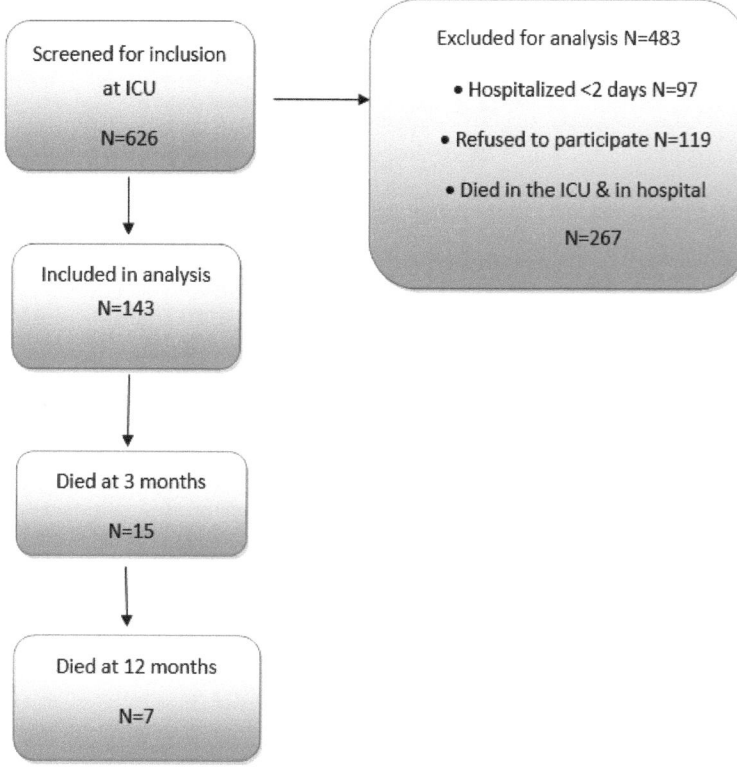

Figure 1. Flow chart of the study.

Figure 2 presents the SF-36 physical and mental health component scores of the participants over 12 months following their hospital discharge. The SF-36 physical scores at hospital discharge, 3 months and 12 months were 27.32 (19.59), 40.97 (26.34) and 50.78 (28.26) ($p < 0.0001$), respectively; the mental health scores at hospital discharge, 3 months and 12 months were 42.93 (17.00), 55.19 (23.04) and 62.24 (23.66) $p < 0.0001$, respectively.

Table 2. Clinical characteristics of participants in the study.

Cause of Admission	
-Medical, n (%)	79 (55.25)
-Pneumonia, n (%)	6 (4.20)
-ARDS, n (%)	10 (6.99)
-Stroke, n (%)	31 (21.6)
Surgical, n (%)	48 (33.56)
APACHE II score	19 (1.1)
Mechanical ventilation, n (%)	126 (88.1)
Mechanical ventilation duration, (median (IQR)), days	5 (2–12)
ICU stay, (median (IQR)), days	7 (3–14)
Hospital Stay, (median (IQR)), days	20 (15–20)
Spirometry *	
FEV1, %pred	69.5 (21.5)
FVC, %pred	69.5 (20.4)
FEVI/FVC, %pred	106 (97–121)
PEF, %pred	58.5 (25.1)
6MWT *, meters	43.84 (28.79)

Data are presented as the mean (SD) unless otherwise indicated. * Values at hospital discharge. ARDS: acute respiratory distress syndrome; FEV1: forced expiratory volume; FVC: forced vital capacity; FEV1/FVC: the ratio of the forced expiratory volume in the first second compared to the forced vital capacity of the lungs; PEF: peak expiratory flow; 6MWT: six-minute walking test.

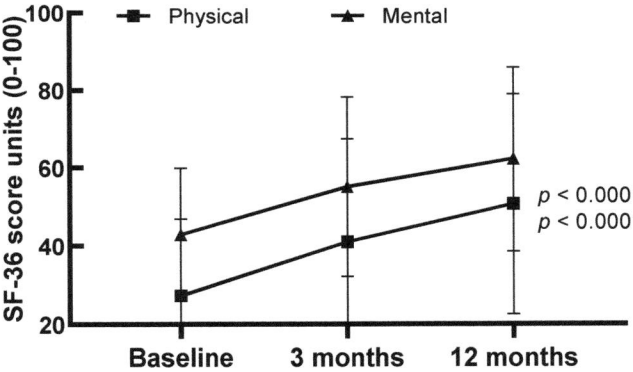

Figure 2. Physical and mental health scores of participants at different time points following ICU discharge. Data are presented as mean (SD) values.

3.1. Lung Function and 6MWT

Lung function in terms of spirometric values and patients' performances in the 6MWT over time are presented in Figure 3 The 6MWT distances (meters) at discharge, 3 months and 12 months were 43.8 (28.8), 59.6 (37.8) and 160.4 (97.5) ($p = 0.0001$), respectively.

The forced expiratory volumes in one second (FEV1) (liters) were 2.20 (0.81), 2.30 (0.92) and 2.40 (0.81), ($p = 0.013$), respectively, and the forced vital capacity (FVC) (liters) was 2.63 (0.96), 2.80 (1.11) and 2.95 (0.93), ($p = 0.023$), respectively.

3.2. Family Support and SF-36 Scores

Figure 4 presents details on daily support at different time points following hospital discharge. One-hundred and forty-two out of one-hundred and forty-three (99.30%) patients received support by one or more family members, one hundred and thirteen (79.02%) by their spouses and eighty-two (42.65%) by one or more friends. Patients received support in their daily activities by their spouses at baseline, 3 months and 12 months for 15.14 h/day, 9.76 h/day and 6.35 h/day ($p < 0.0001$), respectively.

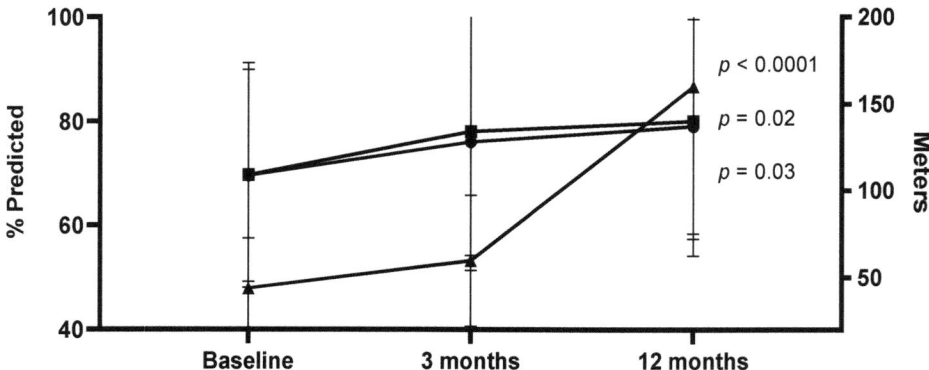

Figure 3. Spirometric values (forced expiratory volume in one second (FEV1) and forced vital capacity (FVC) and the six-minute walking test (6MWT) distances at different time points following ICU discharge. Data are presented as mean (SD) values.

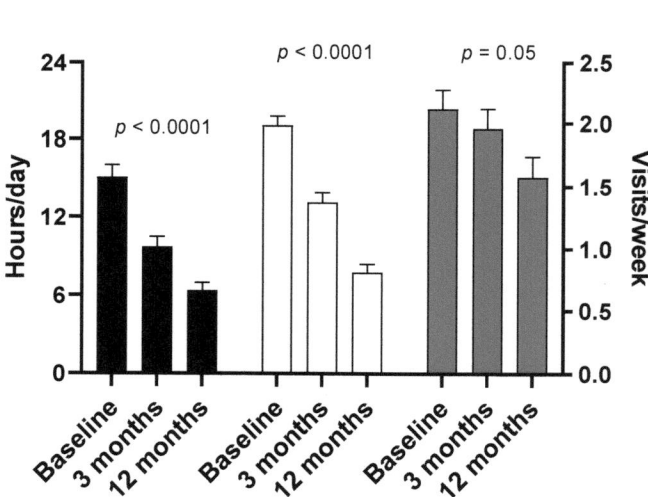

Figure 4. Duration of daily support by family members/spouses (hours/day) and frequency of visits by friends (number of visits/week) to patients at different time points following ICU discharge. Data are presented as mean (SD) values.

Male patients received significantly more frequently support by their family in terms of hours/day compared to females ($p = 0.03$). There was no association between the gender and the number of family members involved in either supportive care or with the duration of support by spouses or with the number of visits by friends. Participants with basic education received significantly more frequent support by their family in terms of hours/day. No other significant association was found between the demographic factors and types of support by family, spouses and friends.

Tables 3 and 4 present patients with improved SF-36 scores ($\geq$median of the relevant score of the total population or not) at 12 months follow-up. Patients with $\geq$median scores had significantly increased lung function compared to patients who presented lower than the median score. Patients with $\geq$median scores presented also shorter ICU stays

(p = 0.0004) and hospital stays (p = 0.014). Those who presented ≥median SF-36 scores at 12 months also had significantly lower frequencies of a stroke at admission (p = 0.001). Participants with ≥median scores were supported more frequently by more than two family members daily or by their friends (more than three times per week).

Table 3. Participant characteristics according to the median value of the physical domain of the SF36 questionnaire at 12 months.

	≥Median SF36 Score N = 71	<Median SF36 Score N = 72	p Value
Age, years	54 (35–69)	66 (52–75)	0.0001
Male, n (%)	43 (60.5)	42 (58.3)	0.6
Stroke, n (%)	7 (9.8)	24 (33.3)	0.0001
ICU stay > 10 days, n (%)	17 (23.9)	36 (50)	0.001
Hospital stay > 10 days, n (%)	58 (81.6)	69 (95.8)	0.001
FEV1, % pred	86 (73–97.7)	49.5 (43.2–54.7)	0.0001
FVC, % pred	81 (68–93)	48 (44–53.5)	0.0001
FEV1/FVC, % pred	104 (95.5–112.5)	46 (43–52)	0.0001
PEF, % pred	81 (69–95)	47 (38–51)	0.0001
6MWT, meters	153 (99–250)	65 (38–101.5)	0.0001
Support by spouses 24/24 h, n (%)	10 (14.0)	12 (16.6)	0.8
Friends' visits > 3/week, n (%)	39 (54.9)	14 (19.4)	0.0001
Family-Support > 2 members, n (%)	61 (85.9)	46 (63.8)	0.001

Data are presented as the median (IQR) unless otherwise indicated. FEV1: forced expiratory volume; FVC: forced vital capacity; FEV1/FVC: the ratio of the forced expiratory volume in the first second compared to the forced vital capacity of the lungs; PEF: peak expiratory flow; 6MWT: the six-minute walking test.

Table 4. Participant characteristics according to the median value of the mental domain of the SF36 questionnaire at 12 months.

	≥Median SF36 Score N = 73	<Median SF36 Score N = 70	p Value
Age, years	54 (36.5–69)	65.5 (53–74)	0.0001
Male, n (%)	45 (61.6)	40 (57.1)	0.9
Stroke, n (%)	7 (9.6)	24 (34.3)	0.001
ICU stay > 10 days, n (%)	19 (26)	39 (55.7)	0.001
Hospital stay > 10 days, n (%)	57 (78)	69 (97.1)	0.002
FEV1, % pred	88 (74–100)	54 (48.5–58.5)	0.0001
FVC, % pred	84 (78–99)	60 (52–65)	0.0001
FEV1/FVC, % pred	104 (95.5–112.5)	46 (43–52)	0.0001
PEF, % pred	88 (78–97)	49 (39.5–55)	0.0001
6MWT, meters	170 (106–250)	36.6 (7.5–58)	0.0001
Support by spouses 24/24 h, n (%)	12 (16.4)	10 (14.3)	0.3
Friends' visits > 3/week, n (%)	36 (49.3)	17 (24.3)	0.001
Family-Support > 2 members, n (%)	60 (82.2)	47 (67.1)	0.003

Data are presented as the median (IQR) unless otherwise indicated. FEV1: forced expiratory volume; FVC: forced vital capacity; FEV1/FVC: the ratio of the forced expiratory volume in the first second compared to the forced vital capacity of the lungs; PEF: peak expiratory flow; 6MWT: the six-minute walking test.

4. Discussion

The main findings of the present study are (a) participants who received more frequent care by more than two members of their families presented better QoL at 3 and 12 months after their discharge from hospital compared to patients who received care by fewer members, (b) participants with ≥median of the SF36 score of the total population at 12 months were supported more frequently by more than two family members daily or by their friends (more than three times per week) compared to patients with <median scores and, (c) similarly, participants with ≥median of the SF36 score of the total population at 12 months had higher values in spirometry or in the 6MWT compared to patients with <median values of the cohort.

The evidence shows that, even years after ICU admission, patients' QoL are significantly decreased compared to the general healthy population [13]. According to Wytske et al. (2021) [14], patients presented several problems both physically and cognitively one year after being admitted to the ICU. The present study assessed the QoL during a 12-month period at three different time points following ICU discharge in a Mediterranean region during the COVID-19 pandemic. Our results suggest that patients recovered gradually in terms of their QoL and presented maximum improvement in their SF-36 scores at twelve months. The SF-36 scores in the physical and mental domains were 45.5 (29.6) and 57.8 (24.7), respectively; these values were significantly higher compared to the respective values at hospital discharge and at the 3-month follow-up. There are no available data for the SF-36 score evolution over time in this setting in Greece. The mean SF score in a population with heart disease in Sweden was 70 [15]. In this respect, one might argue that our population, despite the improvement in QoL at 12 months following ICU, still had compromised QoL at that time point.

Previous studies of the field have suggested that the majority of long-term care for adult patients, either at home or in a community facility, is provided by 90% of their family members [16,17]. The present study shows that patients who were supported more frequently by two or more family members had SF-36 scores at 12 months that were ≥median value of the total cohort compared to patients who were less supported. A plausible explanation might be that the quality of care may be enhanced when many family members are involved in supporting a patient. We speculate that it is possible to provide better help in practical issues (i.e., patients' mobility, enhanced communication and household help) or they may offer psychological support, both important for patients to recover better and faster. Another plausible explanation might be that aged persons have fewer social networks, and therefore, the difference in QoL may be due to age and associated comorbid conditions rather than the presence of social support itself. We believe that a future investigation could define if a specific type of support may be significantly associated with recovery.

Previous studies showed that the relationship between spouses' care and the course of patients' health is important. Spouses may spend long hours every day transferring and helping their spouses who cannot care for themselves. In almost two-thirds of critically ill patients, it is their spouses who cared for them after their discharge from the ICU. Furthermore, younger spouses and females played a more active and regular role in the care of patients compared to elderly or male ones [10,18,19]. In this study, we found that ICU patients present better QoL when their spouses cared for them for more than 8 h daily. In Greece, there are certain deficiencies in the organized distributed support [20] by the state to seriously ill patients when they return to their home environment. It would be of benefit for patients following their discharge from the ICU and hospital to be supported by specialized groups of professionals that can provide home care and can assist spouses and other siblings who live with the critically ill patients.

In this study, we found that the shorter the stay in the ICU for a patient, the better their QoL will be. Previous studies of the field have shown an adverse association between the length of stay in the ICU and the QoL of patients. Notably, when mechanical ventilation (MV) was used for more than seven days, patients manifested worse QoL. In addition, staying in the ICU for more than ten days was associated with higher mortality rates [18]. The contribution of the family is very important in this case as well. Family members' support and visits at the ICU can reduce the length of stay; it has been observed that communication and showing deep love and affection may affect the QoL positively [6,21,22]. In this respect, ICU planning should incorporate the maximum possible support from relatives, when possible, to maximize their benefits and facilitate patients' recovery.

In addition, we found that QoL was associated with the presence of acute neurological illness. Previous studies have shown that stroke is the second leading cause of death and disability worldwide, and depending on the severity of the stroke, it can cause reduced physical fitness and quality of life. The consequences for the reduced QoL of patients suffering from a stroke are related to the duration of stay at the hospital and the program that they followed when discharged [23–26]. These patients cannot be independent, because most of them have permanent disabilities and must change their daily lives. In this respect, they may need support from their family environment for their self-care. Needless to say, the contribution of a specialized staff to help them deal with their problems and improve their health is of crucial importance.

In the present investigation, we assessed patients' physical performances and lung function following the ICU in terms of the 6MWT distance and spirometry. Previous studies have suggested that ICU patients who survived four months after discharge had significantly worse outcomes than the healthy population [27,28]. The 6MWT performance of ICU patients has been studied in severe respiratory disease; ARDS survivors presented significantly reduced 6-min walking distances at six months and one year follow-up [29–31]. In our study, we found improvement in the 6MWT distance at 3 and 12 months after ICU discharge, however, the absolute distances were lower compared to healthy patients who usually present higher 6MWT distances (over 600 m) [28]. It remains elusive whether ICU patients may regain their previous performances over longer time periods. Similar to the 6MWT distance, patients' lung function presented significant improvement over 12 months in our study. Previous investigations showed that patients with ARDS presented mild abnormalities in lung spirometry following the ICU [32–34] or they may have presented fluctuations that were within the normal limits during 3 to 5 years of follow-up.

The present study presents certain limitations that should be taken into consideration when interpreting its findings. First, this is a one-center study that presents data from a specific area in Central Greece, and the sample size of the population studied may be relatively small to evaluate specific subgroups. However, this center provides services to a respectively large population of people, and the results of the study could be useful in implementing strategies at the local level. Moreover, the questionnaire used in the study did not include questions with details on patients' pre-hospital stay or their specific mental support following patients' discharge from hospital. In addition, this study does not provide details related to public and private health support for the patients. This type of support is not standard, and thus, we cannot evaluate its impact on the QoL of patients. Furthermore, the study does not provide details for MV variables in terms of the MV mode, the MV settings used in the ICU or the mechanical properties of the respiratory systems of the participants. We certainly acknowledge that these details may have provided more insight on the evolution of patients' health over time.

5. Conclusions

In conclusion, this observational study suggests that critical care patients presented significant improvement at 12 months following ICU admission in their QoL, lung function and physical performance in terms of the SF-36 assessment, spirometry and 6MWT, respectively. Daily support by family members and frequent visits by friends may have a positive impact on the QoL of critical care patients following their discharge from the hospital.

6. Relevance to Clinical Practice

The role of family members and friends is particularly important for patients after their discharge from the ICU. Family members and friends support during patients' daily activities may help in their recovery and improved quality of life in the long term. The participation of family members could be incorporated into relevant programs that aim to improve patients' recovery from critical illnesses.

Author Contributions: Conceptualization, D.M. and K.A.; Data collection, D.M., K.A., V.T., M.S. and G.F.; Draft preparation D.M. and K.A.; Manuscript review, E.Z., Supervision, D.M. and E.Z. All authors have read and agreed to the published version of the manuscript.

Funding: This research received no external funding.

Institutional Review Board Statement: The study was conducted in accordance with the Declaration of Helsinki and approved by the Institutional Review Board (or Ethics Committee) of University Hospital of Larissa (No. 43704, 1 October 2019).

Informed Consent Statement: Informed consent was obtained from all subjects involved in the study.

Data Availability Statement: Any data related to the study can be provided upon a reasonable request.

Conflicts of Interest: The authors declare no conflict of interest.

References

1. Fernando, A.; Santos, C.; Maia, P.; Maria, A. Castro and Henrique Barros. Quality of life after stay in surgical intensive care unit. *BMC Anesthesiol.* **2007**, *7*, 8.
2. Amy, P.; Bradley, M. Post-intensive care syndrome symptoms and health-related quality of life in family decision-makers of critically ill patients. *Palliat. Support. Care* **2018**, *16*, 719–724.
3. Sidiras, G.; Patsaki, I.; Karatznos, E.; Dakoutrou, M.; Kouvarakos, A.; Mitsiou, G.; Routsi, C.; Stranjalis, G.; Nanas, S.; Gerovasili, V. Long term follow-up of quality of life and functional ability in patients with ICU acquired Weakness-A post hoc analysis. *J. Crit. Care* **2019**, *53*, 223–230. [CrossRef] [PubMed]
4. Vogel, G.; Forinder, U.; Sandgren, A.; Svensen, C.; Joelsson-Alm, E. Health-related quality of life after general surgical intensive care. *Acta Anaesthesiol. Scand.* **2018**, *23*, 1112–1119. [CrossRef] [PubMed]
5. Sarah, E.; Jolley, D.; Aaron, E.; Bunnell, D.; Catherine, L. Icu-acquired weakness. *Chest* **2016**, *150*, 1129–1140.
6. Davidson, E.; Aslakson, A.; Long, C.; Puntillo, A.; Kross, K.; Hart, J.; Cox, E.; Wunsch, H.; Wickline, A.; Nunnally, E.; et al. Guidelines for family-Centered Care in the Neonatal, Pediatric and adult ICU. *Crit. Care Med.* **2017**, *45*, 103–128. [CrossRef]
7. White, B.; Angus, C.; Shields, M.; Buddadhumaruk, R.; Pidro, C.; Paner, C.; Chaitin, E.; Chang, C.; Pike, F.; Weissfeld, L.; et al. A Randomized Trial of a Family-Support Intervention in Intensive Care Units. *N. Engl. J. Med.* **2018**, *378*, 2365–2375. [CrossRef]
8. Davidson, J.E.; Powers, K.; Hedayat, K.M.; Tieszen, M.; Kon, A.A.; Shepard, E.; Spuhler, V.; Todres, I.D.; Levy, M.; Barr, J.; et al. Clinical practice guidelines for support of the family in the patient-centered intensive care unit: American College of Critical Care Medicine Task Force 2004–2005. *Crit. Care Med.* **2007**, *35*, 605–622. [CrossRef]
9. Davidson, E.; Jones, C.; Joseph, O. Family response to critical illness. *Crit. Care Med.* **2012**, *40*, 618–624. [CrossRef]
10. Ashwin, K.; Emily, A.; Diaz-Ramirez, G.; Amy, K.; Ornstein, K.; Boscardin, J.; Smith, A. "Til death do us part": End-of-life experiences of married couples in a nationally representative survey. *J. Am. Geriatr. Soc.* **2018**, *66*, 2360–2366.
11. American Thoracic Society. Standardization of Spirometry, 1994 Update. American Thoracic Society. *Am. J. Respir. Crit. Care Med.* **1995**, *152*, 1107–1136. [CrossRef]
12. American Thoracic Society. ATS statement: Guidelines for the six-minute walk test. *Am. J. Respir. Crit. Care Med.* **2002**, *166*, 111–117. [CrossRef]
13. Soliman, I.; Dylan, W.L.; Peelen, L.; Cremer, L.; Slooter, A.; Pasma, W.; Kesecioglu, J.; Dijk, D. Single-center large-cohort study into quality of life in Dutch intensive care unit subgroups, 1 year after admission, using EuroQoL EQ-6D-3L. *J. Crit. Care* **2015**, *30*, 181–186. [CrossRef] [PubMed]
14. Wytske, W. The Impact of Critical Illness: Long Term Physical, Mental and Cognitive Health Problems in ICU Survivors. 2021. Available online: https://repository.ubn.ru.nl/bitstream/handle/2066/239950/239950.pdf?sequence=1 (accessed on 9 April 2023).
15. Nilsson, E.; Festin, K.; Lowen, M.; Kristenson, M. SF-36 predicts 13-year CHD incidence in a middle-age Swedish general population. *Qual Life Res.* **2020**, *29*, 971–975. [CrossRef]
16. Family Caregiver Alliance Caregiver Assessment: Principles, Guidelines and Strategies for Change. Report from a National Consensus Development Conference. 2006. Available online: https://www.caregiver.org/sites/caregiver.org/files/pdfs/v1consensus.pdf (accessed on 22 January 2023).
17. National Association of Chronic Disease Directors CDC Seeks to Protect Health of Family Caregivers. 2009. Available online: https://cdn.ymaws.com/www.chronicdiseas.org/resource/resmgr/healthy_aging_critical_issues_brief/ha_cib_healthoffamilycaregiv.pdf (accessed on 22 January 2023).
18. Wintermann, G.; Petrowski, K.; Weidner, K.; Straub, B.; Rosendahl, J. Impact of post-traumatic stress symptoms on the health-related quality of life in a cohort study with chronically critically ill patients and their partners: Age matters. *Crit. Care* **2019**, *23*, 39. [CrossRef]
19. Kalavina, R.; Chisati, E.; Mlenzana, N.; Mlenzana, M. The challenges and experiences of stroke patients and their spouses in Blantyre, Malawi. *Wazakili Malawi Med. J.* **2019**, *31*, 112–117. [CrossRef]
20. Mitchell, E.; Moore, K. Stroke: Holistic care and management. *Nurs. Stand.* **2004**, *18*, 43–52. [CrossRef] [PubMed]
21. Hege, H.; Regina, E.; Ingeborg, A.; Tove, P.; Berit, S.; Stine, L.; Gorill, H. From breaking point to breakthrough during the ICU stay: A qualitative study of family members' experiences of long-term intensive care patient' pathway towards survival. *J. Clin. Nurs.* **2018**, *27*, 3630–3640.
22. Barcellos, R.; Chatkin, J. Impact of multidisciplinary checklist on the duration of invasive mechanical ventilation and length of ICU stay. *J. Bras. Pneumol.* **2020**, *46*, 1806–3756. [CrossRef]

23. Henrique, N.; Queiros, P. Patient with stroke: Hospital discharge planning, functionality and quality of life. *Rev. Bras. Enferm.* **2017**, *70*, 415–423.
24. Mohamed, D.; Hashem, N.; Swaroopa, N.; Krishidhar, N.; Nausran, U.; Robinson, K.; Dinglas, V.; Needham, D.; Michelle, N. Eakin Patients' outcomes after critical illness: A systematic review of qualitative studies following hospital discharge. *Crit. Care* **2016**, *20*, 345.
25. Chun, P.; Yip, P.; Tai, J.; Lou, F. Needs of family caregivers of stroke patients: A longitudinal study of caregivers' perspectives. *Patient Prefer. Adherence* **2015**, *9*, 449–457.
26. Tran, P.; Mannen, J. Improving oral healthcare: Improving the quality of life for patients after a stroke. *Spec. Care Dent.* **2009**, *29*, 218–221. [CrossRef] [PubMed]
27. Regis, R.; Dietrich, C.; Valle, T.; Denise, S.; Tagliari, L.; Mattioni, M.; Tonietto, F.; Rosa, R.; Barbosa, G.; Lovatel, G.; et al. The 6-Minute Walk test predicts long-term physical improvement among intensive care unit survivors: A prosective study. *Rev. Bras. Ter. Intensiv.* **2021**, *33*, 374–383.
28. Halliday, S.; Wang, L.; Yu, C.; Vickers, B.; Newman, J.; Fremont, R.; Huerta, L.; Brittain, E.; Hemnes, A. Six-minute walk distance in healthy young adults. *Respir. Med.* **2020**, *165*, 105933. [CrossRef]
29. Herridge, M.S.; Tansey, C.M.; Matté, A.; Tomlinson, G.; Diaz-Granados, N.; Cooper, A.; Guest, C.B.; Mazer, C.D.; Mehta, S.; Stewart, T.E.; et al. Functional disability 5 years after acute respiratory distress syndrome. *N. Engl. J. Med.* **2011**, *364*, 1293–1304. [CrossRef]
30. Ferrand, N.; Zaouter, C.; Chastel, B.; Dewitte, A.; Ouattara, A.; Fleureau, C.; Roze, H. Health related quality of life and predictive factors six months after intensive care unit discharge. *Anaesth. Crit. Care Pain Med.* **2019**, *38*, 137–141. [CrossRef]
31. Kattainanen, S.; Lindahl, A.; Vasankari, T.; Ollila, H.; Volmonen, K.; Piirila, P.; Kauppi, P.; Paajanen, J.; Kreivi, R.; Ulenius, L.; et al. Lung function and exersice capacity 6 months after hospital discharge for critical COVID-19. *BMC Pulm. Med.* **2022**, *22*, 243.
32. Heyland, D.; Groll, D.; Caeser, M. Survivors of acute respiratory distress syndrome: Relationship between pulmonary dysfuction and long-term health-related quality of life. *Crit. Care Med.* **2005**, *33*, 1549–1556. [CrossRef]
33. Rabe, K.F.; Hurd, S.; Anzueto, A.; Barnes, P.J.; Buist, S.A.; Calverley, P.; Zielinski, J. Global strategy for the diagnosis, management and prevention of chronic obstructive pulmonary disease: Gold executive summary. *Am. Respir. Care Med.* **2007**, *176*, 532–555. [CrossRef] [PubMed]
34. Shuai, S.; Hanyujie, K.; Zhenbei, Q.; Yingquan, W.; Zhaohui, T. Effect of different levels of PEEP on mortality in ICU patients without acute respiratory distress syndrome: Systematic review and meta-analysis with trial sequential analysis. *J. Crit. Care* **2021**, *65*, 246–258.

Disclaimer/Publisher's Note: The statements, opinions and data contained in all publications are solely those of the individual author(s) and contributor(s) and not of MDPI and/or the editor(s). MDPI and/or the editor(s) disclaim responsibility for any injury to people or property resulting from any ideas, methods, instructions or products referred to in the content.

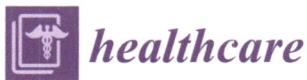

Article

Agreement between Family Members and the Physician's View in the ICU Environment: Personal Experience as a Factor Influencing Attitudes towards Corresponding Hypothetical Situations

Paraskevi Stamou [1], Dimitrios Tsartsalis [2], Georgios Papathanakos [1], Elena Dragioti [3,4,*], Mary Gouva [4] and Vasilios Koulouras [1]

1. Intensive Care Unit, University Hospital of Ioannina, University of Ioannina, 45500 Ioannina, Greece
2. Department of Emergency Medicine, "Hippokration" Hospital, 11527 Athens, Greece
3. Pain and Rehabilitation Centre, Department of Health, Medicine and Caring Sciences, Linköping University, SE-581 83 Linköping, Sweden
4. Laboratory of Psychology of Patients, Families & Health Professionals, Department of Nursing, School of Health Sciences, University of Ioannina, 45500 Ioannina, Greece
* Correspondence: elena.dragioti@liu.se

Abstract: Background: It is not known whether intensive care unit (ICU) patients' family members realistically assess patients' health status. Objectives: The aim was to investigate the agreement between family and intensivists' assessment concerning changes in patient health, focusing on family members' resilience and their perceptions of decision making. Methods: For each ICU patient, withdrawal criteria were assessed by intensivists while family members assessed the patient's health development and completed the Connor–Davidson Resilience Scale and the Self-Compassion Scale. Six months after ICU discharge, follow-up contact was established, and family members gave their responses to two hypothetical scenarios. Results: 162 ICU patients and 189 family members were recruited. Intensivists' decisions about whether a patient met the withdrawal criteria had 75,9% accuracy for prediction of survival. Families' assessments were statistically independent of intensivists' opinions, and resilience had a significant positive effect on the probability of agreement with intensivists. Six months after discharge, family members whose relatives were still alive were significantly more likely to consider that the family or patient themselves should be involved in decision-making. Conclusions: Resilience is related to an enhanced probability of agreement of the family with intensivists' perceptions of patients' health progression. Family attitudes in hypothetical scenarios were found to be significantly affected by the patient's actual health progression.

Keywords: intensive care unit; resilience; realism; family; withdrawal decision

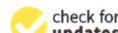

Citation: Stamou, P.; Tsartsalis, D.; Papathanakos, G.; Dragioti, E.; Gouva, M.; Koulouras, V. Agreement between Family Members and the Physician's View in the ICU Environment: Personal Experience as a Factor Influencing Attitudes towards Corresponding Hypothetical Situations. *Healthcare* 2023, 11, 345. https://doi.org/10.3390/healthcare11030345

Academic Editor: Christina Alexopoulou

Received: 6 January 2023
Revised: 20 January 2023
Accepted: 21 January 2023
Published: 25 January 2023

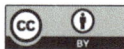

Copyright: © 2023 by the authors. Licensee MDPI, Basel, Switzerland. This article is an open access article distributed under the terms and conditions of the Creative Commons Attribution (CC BY) license (https://creativecommons.org/licenses/by/4.0/).

1. Introduction

Intensive care units (ICUs) are for patients with medical conditions that imminently threaten their survival. Being hospitalized in ICU means that the patient's physical health has suffered excessive and possibly irreversible damage [1]. Additionally, the generally unexpected admission of a patient to the ICU can be particularly frightening and distressing for their loved ones [2]. Higher levels of anxiety, depression, and stress during admission are commonly reported in the literature [3], while post-traumatic stress disorder and complicated grief occur after discharge [4]. Nonetheless, family members are seen as an integral part of the healthcare process and the need for good collaboration should always be considered.

The most important decision made during an ICU stay is often whether to use life-support devices to prolong life, or to discontinue life support and place more emphasis on comfort measures, given that further intervention is futile [5]. To make such a decision as objectively as possible, intensivists have been extensively and thoroughly trained to ensure that their judgment is based on globally recognized health indicators that objectively determine the patient's clinical picture.

Under these circumstances, it is common for the patients not to be able to express their wishes to the medical team [6]. The role of family members is very important, as they are called upon not to express their own opinion on whether the patient's life should be further mechanically assisted, but the patient's own view, based on their perception of the patient's personality and character, or after relevant discussions with the patient prior to admission to the ICU. It is not clearly known whether patients' relatives realistically assess the patient's status of health [6,7]. In fact, an unrealistic perception of the patient's condition on the part of loved ones leads to tension and feelings of unease about the decision to withdraw life support, reflected in overall satisfaction with healthcare system performance [3,8,9].

Moreover, little is known about the factors that influence the patient's family members when asked to make end-of-life decisions on the patient's behalf. In this context, the concepts of mental resilience and self-compassion have been implicated as potential factors in the psychological well-being of families in the ICU, including the subject's ability to succeed despite the adversities they face in life [10] and the subject's ability to have a warm, caring, empathetic, and non-judgmental orientation towards the self at times of suffering and failure [11,12]. Specifically, our group found that self-compassion and mental resilience were highlighted as the two psychological traits that explain the overall psychological distress experienced by attendants in the ICU environment [13].

It is essential to examine the factors influencing the realistic view formed by the patient's relatives, because these directly relate to the quality of communication with medical staff and the overall experience in the ICU. Therefore, the question arises whether these two characteristics are also related to the attendant's increased ability to assess realistically the patient's state of health and to agree with the intensivist's opinion.

A primary aim of the present study was to fill this research gap by examining whether demographic variables, resilience, and self-compassion also influence family members' realistic view of the patients' health. Then, we considered the post-ICU attitudes of family members, and examined whether realistic attitudes during the experienced situation were related to the belief that the family should participate in decision-making in other hypothetical situations, and whether the evolution of the patient's health played an important role. In doing so, we also assessed the validity of hypothetical scenarios as tools for identifying attitudes and perceptions, and their usefulness as policy-making tools.

2. Materials and Methods

2.1. Participants and Study Design

A cross-sectional study was conducted using a quantitative methodology, to evaluate psychological impact on relatives of critically ill patients. The data were collected in two time periods from 2019 to 2021; the first took place during the patient's hospitalization in the ICU of our tertiary university hospital, while the second took place six months after the patient's ICU discharge.

A total of 162 patients and their 189 family members, i.e., spouse, child, parent, or other, were recruited and agreed to participated in the study. Family members of patients with elective postoperative admission or brain death or who died within 1 week after admission were excluded from the study. Oral informed consent was obtained from family members and the study was approved by the Ethics Committee of the University Hospital of Ioannina.

Within the first two days after patient admission, the Glasgow coma score (GSC), the acute physiology, age and chronic health evaluation score (APACHE), and the simplified acute physiology score (SAPS) were assessed by ICU physicians. When the medical status and the prognosis of the patient were clarified, the director of the department together with the 3 most experienced intensivists completed a brief screening questionnaire describing whether the patient met any of eight criteria for withdrawal of treatment, along with a single direct question as to whether the patient would eventually survive. Then, 7–10 days after patient's admission to the ICU and in the knowledge of the intensivists's assessment of the patient's health status, the relatives were asked to complete a multiple-choice questionnaire. For each family member, gender, age, type of relationship, and their assessment of the health progression of their relative were recorded on a five-point Likert scale (1: hopeless to 5: hopeful).

Additionally, each family member completed the Connor–Davidson resilience scale (CD-RISC) [14] and the self-compassion scale (SCS) [12]. The CD-RISC consists of 25 items that are answered on a 5-point frequency scale (0 to 4). CD-RISC's total score ranges from 0 to 100, with higher scores indicating greater perceived resilience [14]. The SCS consists of 26 questions answered on a 5-point frequency scale (1 to 5), and the total score is calculated as the overall mean after 13 of the score values are reversed [12]. The total score reflects self-compassion as defined as a dynamic balance between compassionate and uncompassionate ways in which individuals respond emotionally to pain and failure, cognitively understand their predicament, and pay attention to suffering [12].

Six months after each patient's ICU discharge, telephone follow-up contact was established with 153/189 (81%) of participants, all of whom had close contacts with a patient. During this telephone interview, family members answered four questions about two hypothetical clinical scenarios: one with a conscious and competent patient being able to comprehend his actual state of health, and one with an unconscious patient who cannot participate in medical decisions that affecting him. In both scenarios, the first question assessed whether the patient's family should be involved in the decision to withdraw life support measures, while the second question aimed to capture the family member's opinion about who should be responsible for making the decision. The two scenarios were taken from a previous study [15] and translated into Greek with minor changes in the responses, allowing independent selection of all those involved in the decision-making process.

2.2. Statistical Analysis

The Chi-square test of independence was applied to evaluate whether two nominal or ordinal variables were statistically independent. Analysis of variance was applied to quantify the differences between more than two groups, while Tukey's b test was employed to highlight the homogeneous groups. To elucidate the similarities between respondents' answers in the hypothetical scenarios, the distances between pairs of binary variables were computed using the Dice coefficient of similarity (known also as the Czekanowski or Sorensen measure) [16]. Then, a hierarchical cluster analysis was applied to provide an indicative grouping of similar responses. A logistic regression model was applied to test whether demographic factors, resilience, and self-compassion affected agreement between family members' and intensivists' assessments, and a second logistic model was applied in order to test whether agreement in assessment and the progression of patient's health affected respondents' perceptions in analogous scenarios.

A two-sided level of significance of 0.05 was set for all statistical tests. The data were analyzed using SPSS statistical package (version 21) and R statistical language [17].

3. Results

3.1. Sample Characteristics

The demographic sample characteristics for family members and patients are presented in Table 1. The mean age of family members was 46.5 (SD 11.4 years) and the corresponding figure for the patients was 64.4 (SD 17.2 years). Among the family members, 111 (58.7%) were women; the corresponding figure for the patients was 52 (32.1%).

Table 1. Family members' and patients' characteristics.

Family Members' Characteristics (N = 189)	Mean (SD)
Age	46.5 (11.4)
Gender	Frequency (%)
Women	111 (58.7%)
Men	78 (41.3%)
Type of relation	
Spouse/partner	36 (19%)
Child	97 (51.3%)
Parent	14 (7.4%)
Other	42 (22.2%)
Stay with the patient	77 (40.7%)
Patients' characteristics (n = 162)	Mean (SD)
Age	64.4 (17.2)
Gender	Frequency (%)
Women	52 (32.1%)
Men	110 (67.8%)

N = sample of the family members, n = sample of patients admitted to ICU.

3.2. Intensivists Criteria for Withdrawing Life-Sustaining Treatment

Among the 162 patients admitted to the ICU, 46 (28.4%) met the intensivists' criteria for treatment withdrawal. Lack of future quality of life and futility of treatment were the dominant clinical assessments. Meanwhile, hospital costs were not regarded as a withdrawal criterion for any patient, while age was considered a criterion for six patients (M = 78.7 years, SD = 3.8) (Table 2).

Table 2. Intensivists' criteria for withdrawal or non-escalation of support measures.

Criteria [1]	Frequency (%) [2]	The Patient Meets the Withdrawal Criteria [3]
Lack of future quality of life	49 (30.2%)	38 (82.6%)
Prolonged lack of quality of life	41 (25.3%)	34 (73.9%)
Futility of treatment	27 (16.7%)	25 (54.3%)
Body pain	19 (11.7%)	19 (41.3%)
Wishes of relatives	9 (5.6%)	9 (19.6%)
Moral pain	6 (3.7%)	6 (13%)
Patient's age	6 (3.7%)	5 (10.9%)
Cost	0 (0%)	0 (0%)

[1] Descending frequency order; [2] Percentage of the total n = 162 patients; [3] Percentage of the 46 patients who were judged to meet the withdrawal criteria.

The 46 patients that met the withdrawal criteria were significantly older (73.3 ± 11.5 vs. 60.9 ± 17.8, $p < 0.001$) than the others, they were characterized by significantly higher SAPS scores (54.7 ± 13.8 vs. 39.1 ± 12.7, $p < 0.001$) and APACHE scores (21.5 ± 5.7 vs. 15.9 ± 5.8, $p < 0.001$), and significantly lower GCS scores (7.0 ± 3.0 vs. 10.1 ± 3.5, $p < 0.001$). During ICU hospitalization, 25/46 passed away, with the remaining 21 patients at ICU discharge presenting severe disability regarding feeding (nasogastric tube or gastrostomy), breathing (tracheostomy), or mobility (hemiplegia, tetraplegia, critical care myopathy). Six months after ICU hospitalization, nine patients were still alive with little (7) or moderate (2) health recovery, and unable to live autonomously. Overall, the accuracy of the physician's classification (PAC) concerning patient's survival was 75.9% during hospitalization, and 71% six months after hospitalization (Table 3).

Table 3. Patients' survival at ICU discharge and 6 months later, and survival prediction.

Time	Patients (n)	Survival	The Patient Met the Withdrawal Criteria		Intensivists' Survival Prediction Indexes		
			No	Yes	Percentageaccuracy [1]	Sensitivity [2]	Specificity [3]
Discharge from ICU	162	119	98	21	75.9%	84.5%	54.3%
After six months	112/119 *	87	78	9	71.0%	67.2%	80.4%

[1] Percentage of patients correctly classified as survivals or non-survivals. [2] Percentage of patients classified as not meeting the survival criteria who subsequently survived. [3] Percent of patients classified as meeting the withdrawal criteria who died. n = sample of patients admitted to ICU. * 6 months after ICU discharge, it was possible to contact family members for 112 out of 119 patients.

3.3. Family Members' Agreement with Intensivists Concerning Patient's Health

About half of the 189 respondents (86, 45.5%) were overly optimistic about the patient's health progress (Table 4). The subjective optimism expressed by the patients' family members was statistically independent of the intensivist's evaluation ($c^2(4) = 6.279$, $p = 0.179$). The family members were divided into three categories according to their assessments, in comparison with the those of the intensivists. The first category comprised family members who did not expect a positive change in the patient's health, while the doctors insisted on the continuation of life support ($N = 38$). The second group contained the family members who perceived the patient's state of health in agreement with the intensivist's perception ($N = 108$), and the third category included family members who expected a positive development in the patient's health while the intensivists suggested withdrawal of life support ($N = 36$). Overall, 74 (40.7%) of the respondents were not in agreement with intensivists' judgments about changes in the health of their relative (Table 4).

Table 4. Family members' assessment of the progress of patient health and comparison to the intensivists' assessment.

Family Member's Assessment about Patient's Health Progression	N (%)	The Corresponding Patient Meets the Withdrawal Criteria (Intensivist's Judgment)		Agreement of Judgment (Family Member's Judgment Compared to Intensivist's)		
		No	Yes	Agree [1]	Not Agree	
					Pessimistic	Optimistic
Hopeless	14 (7.4%)	7	7	7	7	
2	12 (6.3%)	9	3	3	9	
3	29 (15.3%)	22	7		22	7
4	41 (21.7%)	29	12	29		12
Hopeful	86 (45.5%)	69	17	69		17
Total	182 (100%)	136	46	108	38	36

[1] Family member's judgment compared to intensivist's. N = sample of the family members.

The mean resilience score for the total sample of family members was 70.8 (SD = 14.4) analogous to the general Greek population (MP = 70.2, SD = 11.4) [18]. The mean score for self-compassion was 3.3 (SD = 0.5), considered moderate (2.5 to 3.5) due to the lack of clinical norms or scores to suggest that an individual has high or low self-compassion [19].

Logistic regression was carried out to quantify the effects of the patients' age and gender, family members' age and gender, staying with the patient, resilience, and self-compassion in terms of the agreement between the attendant's and intensivist's assessment of the patient's health. The logistic model was statistically significant (omnibus test of model coefficients: $c2(8) = 19.432$, $p = 0.013$), being able to predict correctly 66.7% of the observations (sensitivity 81.6%, specificity 45.1%, 2-log likelihood = -215.865, McFadden's pseudo R squared = 0.083) (Table 5).

The attendant's resilience (B = 0.031, ExpB = 1.032, 95% C.I. 1.005–1.060, $p = 0.022$), had a significant effect on the probability of agreement concerning the patient's health. Specifically, an additional score of one on the resilience scale corresponded to 1.032 times greater likelihood that the respondent agreed with the intensivist's view of the patient's health. In particular, those who agreed were characterized by a significantly higher resilience score (M_{NA} = 68.0 vs. M_{AG} = 73.0, $t(172)$ = 2.402, p = 0.017).

The effect of the patient's age on realism was marginally rejected at the 0.05 level (B = −0.020, ExpB = 0.980, 95% C.I. 0.960–1.000, p = 0.050), suggesting a noteworthy but not significant effect. In this context, it is worth noting that the statistically significant difference between patient age in the two groups (M_{NA} = 68.0 vs. M_{AG} = 60.6, $t(172)$ = 2.775, p = 0.006).

Table 5. Logistic prediction model of agreement between attendants' and intensivists' assessments.

Variable	B	SE	Wald	df	P	Exp B	95% C.I Lower	95% C.I Upper
Intercept	1.005	1.508	0.444	1	0.505	2.731		
Patient's demographic								
Gender	−0.293	0.354	0.683	1	0.408	0.746	0.373	1.494
Age	−0.020	0.010	3.843	1	0.050	0.980	0.960	1.000
Family members' data								
Close relation	−0.424	0.482	0.773	1	0.379	0.654	0.254	1.684
Gender	0.328	0.337	0.948	1	0.330	1.388	0.717	2.688
Age	−0.023	0.015	2.465	1	0.116	0.977	0.949	1.006
Living with the patient	−0.384	0.355	1.170	1	0.279	0.681	0.340	1.366
Resilience	0.031	0.014	5.268	1	0.022	1.032	1.005	1.060
Self-compassion	−0.044	0.373	0.014	1	0.906	0.957	0.461	1.987

3.4. Family Participation in the Theoretical Scenarios, 6 Months after the ICU Experience

At the second sampling timeperiod, among the 153 family members that responded to the study, 13 were parents, 31 were spouses, 18 were brothers, and 91 were offspring. In both hypothetical scenarios, most of the respondents favored family participation in decision making (Scenario 1: 78, 51.0%, Scenario 2: 109, 71.2%) (Table 6).

A logistic regression analysis was applied to test the effects of patient's age, agreement with intensivists during hospitalization, and survival of the patient on the probability of considering family or patient responsible for the withdrawal decision. The logistic model was statistically significant (Omnibus Test of Model Coefficients: c2(5) = 12.888, p = 0.024), being able to predict 66.7% of the observations correctly (sensitivity 93.9%, specificity 18.2%, −2-log likelihood = −186.966, Nagelkerke pseudo R squared = 0.111) (Table 7).

Table 6. The hypothetical clinical scenarios.

Scenario 1	Scenario 2
A 60-year-old married woman with severe cancer and pneumonia needs the assistance of a ventilator in order to breathe. The woman will die within 24 h if the ventilator is withdrawn. The woman's physician is completely convinced that she will die within a period of 1 month regardless of what treatment she receives. The woman is exhausted with her severe disease but fully conscious and able to express her wishes. The intensivists are considering withdrawing the ventilator and allowing her to die, so she will no longer have to suffer.	A 65-year-old married man was in a serious accident in which he suffered head injuries. One month later he is still unconscious and needs the assistance of a ventilator in order to breathe. The man will die within 24 h if the ventilator is withdrawn. The physician is completely convinced that he will not wake up, although he might live for a while if the ventilator is kept in place. The intensivists are considering withdrawing the ventilator treatment and allowing him to die.
Question 1 The intensivistsraise the question of continued ventilator treatment. Who should participate in this discussion? Answers: • The patient, n = 102 (66.7%) • The family, n = 82 (53.6%) • Only the intensivists, n = 13 (8.5%) • Uncertain, n = 12 (7.8%)	*Question 1*: The intensivists raise the question of continued ventilator treatment. Who should participate in this discussion? Answers: • The family, n = 133 (86.9%) • Only the intensivists, n = 17 (11.1%) • Uncertain, n = 20 (13.1%)

Table 6. *Cont.*

Scenario 1	Scenario 2
Question 2: Assuming that the intensivists have brought up the question of ventilator treatment for discussion, whom do you believe should decide whether or not the ventilator treatment should be continued? Answers: • The patient, $n = 106$ (69.3%) • The family, $n = 78$ (51.0%) • Only the intensivist, $n = 78$ (51.0%) • Uncertain, $n = 14$ (9.2%)	*Question 2*: Assuming that the intensivists have brought up the question of ventilator treatment for discussion with the family, whom do you believe should decide whether or not the ventilator treatment should be continued? Answers: • The family, $n = 109$ (71.2%) • Only the intensivist, $n = 89$ (58.2%) • Uncertain, $n = 21$ (13.7%) • The treatment should not be stopped, $n = 12$ (7.8%)

n = groups of answers within the total sample.

Table 7. Effects of patients' characteristics on family/patient selection in the two theoretical scenarios.

Variable	B	SE	Wald	df	p	Exp B	95% C.I Lower	95% C.I Upper
Intercept	−0.075	0.972	0.006	1	0.939	0.928		
Agree with intensivists during hospitalization	0.584	0.393	2.215	1	0.137	1.794	0.831	3.872
Health Condition			5.118	2	0.077			
Not autonomous vs. Deceased	−4.892	2.769	3.122	1	0.077	0.008	0.000	1.707
Autonomous vs. Deceased	−5.319	2.360	5.079	1	0.024	0.005	0.000	0.500
Age	0.015	0.015	0.988	1	0.320	1.015	0.986	1.044
Age × Condition			6.873	2	0.032			
Not autonomous vs. Deceased	0.068	0.041	2.820	1	0.093	1.071	0.989	1.159
Autonomous vs. Deceased	0.088	0.034	6.864	1	0.009	1.092	1.022	1.166

A significant interaction between the patient's age and his or her health condition was identified (Wald W = 6.873, df = 2, $p = 0.032$). Specifically, as the age of patients increased, respondents whose relatives were still alive and lived autonomously were significantly more likely to consider the patient himself or the family as those who should be involved in decision making. In contrast, in cases where the patient had died, as the age of their deceased relatives increased the respondents tended to hesitate to declare the family responsible for decision making in the theoretical scenarios (Figure 1).

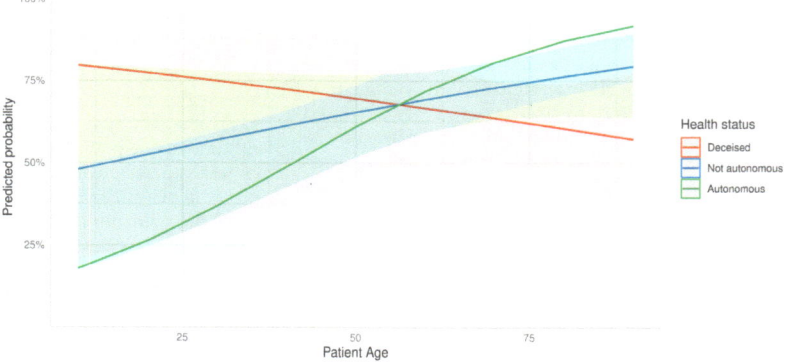

Figure 1. Interaction effect of age and health status on family members' selections in the hypothetical scenarios. Predicted probability refers to the probability of a response that the patient himself or the family should be involved in the decision-making.

4. Discussion

Withdrawal of life-sustaining therapy, while not a strictly documented procedure, is an ethically acceptable practice in western ICUs. For example, in the Ethicus-2 study, a prospective observational study of 199 ICUs in 36 countries involving 87,951 patients who were admitted to ICU over a 6-month period, 12,850 (14.6%) patients died, with treatment limitations (withholding or withdrawing life-sustaining treatment) occurring frequently (80.9%). Common factors associated with treatment limitation included patient's age and chronic disease, together with the presence of country-specific end-of-life legislation [20,21]. The decision to withdraw extensive supportive care is made by ICU physicians, based on measurable indicators of physical functioning and objective observations of vital signs. As most critically ill patients lack decision-making capacity and family members often serve as surrogate decision makers, decisions about the end of life should involve the family. Unfortunately, not only do data about true family participation in end-of-life decisions remain scarce, but end-of-life communication with families or surrogates varies markedly in different global regions; according to the Ethicus-2 study, discussion with family occurred only in 46.4% of cases in southern Europe, while in northern and central Europe percentages were significantly higher at 95.0% and 74.9.%, respectively [22,23]. For Greece, data are even more limited. In a national Greek study conducted across 18 multidisciplinary Greek ICUs dating back to 2015, 71.4% of 149 doctors and 59.8% of 320 nurses responded that families were not actively involved in discussion of life-sustaining treatment, confirming that in Greece fear of litigation is still considered a major barrier to properly informing the patients' relatives about end-of-life decisions [24]. Since no clear, discontinuation criteria are defined in other countries either, the final decision always lies with the physicians, and is usually based on their experience and training [25]. However, making life-or-death decisions for another person is never an inconsequential decision for physicians, as reflected in increased burnout and distress among medical staff [26] and less empathetic and more cynical behaviour towards ICU patients [27]. In this regard, the present study suggests that the psychological pressure faced by medical staff does not affect their assessment of whether patients meet the withdrawal criteria. Poor quality of life in future and futility of treatment were found to be the most important criteria for the discontinuation of life-sustaining measures, while patients' gender or age as well as treatment costs did not significantly influence the decision. It was also found that ICU physician assessment accurately assesses patients' chances of survival during their hospital stay and in the immediate future. It is worth mentioning that in the Ethicus-2 study, 20% of patients with treatment limitations eventually survived the hospital stay, and the percentage in the earlier Ethicus-1 study (1999–2000) was even lower [20,21].

On a different note, in the burdensome environment of an ICU, members of the patient's family are in a vulnerable position where depressive symptoms [28,29] and higher risk of anxiety and stress-related disorders are commonly reported [30]. Given this great psychological pressure, it is not surprising that for out of ten family members did not realistically assess the health progression of their relatives in ICU. In particular, the fact that the psychological symptoms of the family members were independent of the severity of the patient's condition is supported by the findings of previous research [31].

Nevertheless, a realistic view is always necessary, because unjustified optimism makes it difficult to adjust to the loss of a loved one, promotes feelings of meaninglessness, and can lead to painful after-experiences in the ICU. This was demonstrated in the study by Sjökvist et al. [15], where the general public stated that they preferred greater influence from patients and families compared with intensive-care physicians in decisions to withdraw life support. The results of the present study further clarify these differences by highlighting mental resilience as the trait that determines the consent of family members to intensivists' assessments. That is, this study further demonstrates the importance of resilience, previously shown in the study by Stamou et al. [13], as a psychological trait that reduces the overall psychological burden of ICU attendants.

Moreover, resilience, as commonly defined as the process of adapting well in the face of adversity, trauma, tragedy, threats, or significant sources of stress, is highlighted as a key feature facilitating the transition from the initial emotional distress experienced by family members in the ICU to a sense of regained control [13]. As one such key feature, resilience provides family members with the right conditions to seek and create meaning in their situation and gives them purpose in contributing to their relative's recovery. Therefore, an appropriate collaborative approach should be developed between family members and healthcare professionals, to address the patient's needs while providing emotional and psychosocial support to their families [32]. Specifically, it is suggested that initiatives aiming to strengthen mental resilience will help relatives' agreement with the opinions of critical care physicians, enhance quality of communication, reduce feelings of frustration and dissatisfaction from intensivists as well as relatives, and improve the overall satisfaction of the patient's companions about the care their loved one receives [33,34].

After hospitalization in the ICU, most surviving patients require constant and long-term care and are unable to care for themselves. This situation, commonly referred to as post-intensive care syndrome (PICS), can affect the patient's body, thoughts, feelings, and mental state [35]. Of course, this also puts strain on the family environment, both psychologically and financially. In the context of the two theoretical scenarios, caregivers of a surviving patient were reluctant to attribute family responsibility for life-sustaining decisions as their patients aged, a finding that indicates that their personal experiences strongly influenced the responses to the theoretical scenarios. It might be argued that positive health progress appears to predispose respondents to family involvement, while poor progress or the death of a loved one appears to reduce the desire to involve the family in life-support decisions affecting the ICU patient. Overall, a biased attitude was evident in our study, with personal experiences strongly influencing responses to theoretical scenarios. We found that the death of the patient distances the caregiving relative from the traumatic event of their family member's hospitalization in the ICU. Furthermore, results indicated a limited validity of these instruments as decision-making aids with regard to the involvement of the family in withdrawal decisions in the ICU environment.

There is ample evidence in the current literature that family members desire a more active role in end-of-life decision-making, in order to communicate patient's wishes [36]. There is also consensus that end-of-life decisions should be viewed as shared decisions, with shared responsibility between the care team, the patient, and the family [37]. In this context, it is of paramount importance for intensivists to provide patients and their families with reliable information to help them decide whether withdrawal of life-support measures is the appropriate medical option [38]. Complete and comprehensible information about the medical data supporting the discontinuation of patient support could help loved ones to resolve their doubts about the treatment being offered, to understand the futility of the treatment, and to appreciate the severely reduced quality of life that awaits the patient if they survive after ICU [39]. Although the crucial need for complete and accurate information for family members of ICU patients has been widely reported [40,41] this factor seems to be underestimated by caregivers [42]. Since treatment futility is a rather vague concept and various attempts have been made to resolve this problem [43–45], there is a need for improvement in the communication skills of ICU staff so they can better distinguish and describe to relatives the individual aspects of treatment futility. With regard to the goal of family consent to the doctors' decisions, an additional initiator could be the family's right to additional patient care, which has also been described in the literature as a demand [44]. This opportunity would allow family members to experience the situation, recognize the futility of treatment, and create personal meaning for the potential loss of their loved one, making the loss gentler for them. Especially in the current context of COVID-19 with the noted shortage of ICU beds worldwide, better communication skills and methods between family members and caregivers will enable faster decisions and allow medical staff to provide medical care and hospitalization to people who need it most [45,46].

To the best of our knowledge, this is the first study to examine personal experience and resilience in relation to family members' realistic views of ICU patient health as factors influencing attitudes towards end-of-life decisions. The use of disease severity scores such as GSC, APACHE, and SAPS to compare against family views is one of this study's strengths.

Our study had some limitations. First, our results reported responses from one single ICU; hence their lack of generalizability should not be ignored. Second, family members who declined to participate at the second phase of the study i.e., six months after the ICU experience, may have reported different attitudes and perceptions. Furthermore, we did not assess post-ICU distress symptoms or post-ICU resilience and are therefore unable to justify the role played by such factors in long-term attitudes towards end-of-life decisions. Finally, since the data for the hypothetical scenarios were collected six months after ICU experience, the possibility of recall bias cannot be ruled out.

5. Conclusions

Family members of patients admitted to ICU have increased needs in terms of assurance, proximity, and information, and these requirements should be carefully considered by ICU staff [2]. The results of our study indicate that resilience as a personality trait was associated with an increased likelihood of agreement between family members and physicians' perceptions of the patient's health. Thus, it is suggested that mental resilience initiatives can help family members to adapt well to the overwhelming experiences in ICU and to recognize the situation pragmatically. In particular, the development of a philosophy of family-centred care should be a priority, with formal assessment of families taking place shortly after admission, followed by development of an appropriate care plan [47]. From this perspective, a collaborative approach between family members and medical staff will enhance the quality of communication, reduce feelings of frustration and dissatisfaction among physicians and relatives, and improve overall satisfaction with the care received.

Furthermore, family members' perceptions of the patient's health progress are related to their psychological characteristics, while the way they responded to the two hypothetical scenarios was related to their patient's health progress (Supplementary Table S1). Therefore, it is cautioned that family members may have difficulty separating what they feel is best from what they believe the patient would think best [48]. It is suggested that the involvement of family members in important decisions regarding the patient life-support should be required of physicians working in critical care, while it appears that the ultimate decision should remain the sole responsibility of medical staff. However, we believe our findings merit further investigation with increased consideration given to the communication skills between ICU staff and family members; a factor that we did not examine herein.

Finally, the appropriateness of hypothetical scenarios for ascertaining citizens' perceptions is not supported, or at least their more cautious use and careful interpretation of the responses is suggested, which should consider the respondents' recent exposure to relevant traumatic events as well as the trajectory of these events.

Supplementary Materials: The following supporting information can be downloaded at: https://www.mdpi.com/article/10.3390/healthcare11030345/s1. Supplementary Table S1: Proximity matrix of the answers to the four questions in the two hypothetical scenarios (Dice measure).

Author Contributions: Conceptualization, V.K, M.G. and P.S.; methodology, V.K., G.P. and E.D; software, M.G. and E.D.; validation, V.K., G.P. and D.T.; investigation, P.S.; writing—original draft preparation, P.S., D.T and E.D.; writing—review and editing, V.K., G.P. and M.G.; visualization, M.G. and E.D.; supervision, V.K. All authors have read and agreed to the published version of the manuscript.

Funding: This research received no external funding.

Institutional Review Board Statement: The study was conducted in accordance with the Declaration of Helsinki and approved by the Ethics Committee of the University Hospital of Ioannina (protocol code 3263, 1 February 2019).

Informed Consent Statement: Oral informed consent was obtained from all subjects involved in the study.

Data Availability Statement: Not applicable.

Acknowledgments: Naum Konstantina and Evaggelos Ioannou for administrative support.

Conflicts of Interest: The authors declare no conflict of interest.

References

1. Maki, D.G.; Crnich, C.J.; Safdar, N. Nosocomial Infection in the Intensive Care Unit. In *Critical Care Medicine*; Elsevier: Amsterdam, The Netherlands, 2008; pp. 1003–1069. [CrossRef]
2. Alsharari, A.F. The needs of family members of patients admitted to the intensive care unit. *Patient Prefer. Adherence* **2019**, *13*, 465–473. [CrossRef] [PubMed]
3. Abdul Halain, A.; Tang, L.Y.; Chong, M.C.; Ibrahim, N.A.; Abdullah, K.L. Psychological distress among the family members of Intensive Care Unit (ICU) patients: A scoping review. *J. Clin. Nurs.* **2022**, *31*, 497–507. [CrossRef] [PubMed]
4. Cameron, J.I.; Chu, L.M.; Matte, A.; Tomlinson, G.; Chan, L.; Thomas, C.; Friedrich, J.O.; Mehta, S.; Lamontagne, F.; Levasseur, M.; et al. One-Year Outcomes in Caregivers of Critically Ill Patients. *N. Engl. J. Med.* **2016**, *374*, 1831–1841. [CrossRef] [PubMed]
5. Myatra, S.N.; Salins, N.; Iyer, S.; Macaden, S.C.; Divatia, J.V.; Muckaden, M.; Kulkarni, P.; Simha, S.; Mani, R.K. End-of-life care policy: An integrated care plan for the dying: A Joint Position Statement of the Indian Society of Critical Care Medicine (ISCCM) and the Indian Association of Palliative Care (IAPC). *Indian J. Crit. Care Med.* **2014**, *18*, 615–635. [CrossRef]
6. Adams, J.A.; Anderson, R.A.; Docherty, S.L.; Tulsky, J.A.; Steinhauser, K.E.; Bailey, D.E., Jr. Nursing strategies to support family members of ICU patients at high risk of dying. *Heart Lung* **2014**, *43*, 406–415. [CrossRef] [PubMed]
7. Akdeniz, M.; Yardımcı, B.; Kavukcu, E. Ethical considerations at the end-of-life care. *SAGE Open Med.* **2021**, *9*, 20503121211000918. [CrossRef]
8. McAdam, J.L.; Puntillo, K. Symptoms experienced by family members of patients in intensive care units. *Am. J. Crit. Care* **2009**, *18*, 200–209, quiz 210. [CrossRef]
9. Myhren, H.; Ekeberg, Ø.; Stokland, O. Satisfaction with communication in ICU patients and relatives: Comparisons with medical staffs' expectations and the relationship with psychological distress. *Patient Educ. Couns.* **2011**, *85*, 237–244. [CrossRef]
10. Bonanno, G.A. Loss, trauma, and human resilience: Have we underestimated the human capacity to thrive after extremely aversive events? *Am. Psychol.* **2004**, *59*, 20–28. [CrossRef]
11. Gilbert, P. *The Compassionate Mind*; Robinson: Torrance, CA, USA, 2009.
12. Neff, K.D. The Development and Validation of a Scale to Measure Self-Compassion. *Self Identity* **2003**, *2*, 223–250. [CrossRef]
13. Stamou, P.; Gouva, M.; Konstanti, Z.; Papathanasiou, A.; Koulouras, V.; Papathanakos, G. Psychological Factors Affecting the Family's Satisfaction of Patients in an Intensive Care Unit: The Dominant Role of Self-Compassion and Resilience. *Open J. Nurs.* **2022**, *12*, 334–348. [CrossRef]
14. Connor, K.M.; Davidson, J.R. Development of a new resilience scale: The Connor-Davidson Resilience Scale (CD-RISC). *Depress. Anxiety* **2003**, *18*, 76–82. [CrossRef] [PubMed]
15. Sjökvist, P.; Nilstun, T.; Svantesson, M.; Berggren, L. Withdrawal of life support–who should decide? Differences in attitudes among the general public, nurses and physicians. *Intensive Care Med.* **1999**, *25*, 949–954. [CrossRef] [PubMed]
16. Dice, L.R. Measures of the Amount of Ecologic Association Between Species. *Ecology* **1945**, *26*, 297–302. [CrossRef]
17. RC Team. *Core. R: A Language and Environment for Statistical Computing*; RC Team: Vienna, Austria, 2018.
18. Tsigkaropoulou, E.; Douzenis, A.; Tsitas, N.; Ferentinos, P.; Liappas, I.; Michopoulos, I. Greek Version of the Connor-Davidson Resilience Scale: Psychometric Properties in a Sample of 546 Subjects. *In Vivo* **2018**, *32*, 1629–1634. [CrossRef]
19. Neff, K.D. Self-Compassion: Theory, Method, Research, and Intervention. *Annu. Rev. Psychol.* **2023**, *74*, 193–218. [CrossRef]
20. Avidan, A.; Sprung, C.L.; Schefold, J.C.; Ricou, B.; Hartog, C.S.; Nates, J.L.; Jaschinski, U.; Lobo, S.M.; Joynt, G.M.; Lesieur, O.; et al. Variations in end-of-life practices in intensive care units worldwide (Ethicus-2): A prospective observational study. *Lancet Respir. Med.* **2021**, *9*, 1101–1110. [CrossRef]
21. Sprung, C.L.; Cohen, S.L.; Sjokvist, P.; Baras, M.; Bulow, H.H.; Hovilehto, S.; Ledoux, D.; Lippert, A.; Maia, P.; Phelan, D.; et al. End-of-life practices in European intensive care units: The Ethicus Study. *Jama* **2003**, *290*, 790–797. [CrossRef]
22. Hartog, C.S.; Maia, P.A.; Ricou, B.; Danbury, C.; Galarza, L.; Schefold, J.C.; Soreide, E.; Bocci, M.G.; Pohrt, A.; Sprung, C.L.; et al. Changes in communication of end-of-life decisions in European ICUs from 1999 to 2016 (Ethicus-2)—A prospective observational study. *J. Crit. Care* **2022**, *68*, 83–88. [CrossRef]
23. Feldman, C.; Sprung, C.L.; Mentzelopoulos, S.D.; Pohrt, A.; Hartog, C.S.; Danbury, C.; Weiss, M.; Avidan, A.; Estella, A.; Joynt, G.M.; et al. Global Comparison of Communication of End-of-Life Decisions in the ICU. *Chest* **2022**, *162*, 1074–1085. [CrossRef]
24. Ntantana, A.; Matamis, D.; Savvidou, S.; Marmanidou, K.; Giannakou, M.; Gouva, M.; Nakos, G.; Koulouras, V. The impact of healthcare professionals' personality and religious beliefs on the decisions to forego life sustaining treatments: An observational, multicentre, cross-sectional study in Greek intensive care units. *BMJ Open* **2017**, *7*, e013916. [CrossRef]

25. Phua, J.; Joynt, G.M.; Nishimura, M.; Deng, Y.; Myatra, S.N.; Chan, Y.H.; Binh, N.G.; Tan, C.C.; Faruq, M.O.; Arabi, Y.M.; et al. Withholding and withdrawal of life-sustaining treatments in intensive care units in Asia. *JAMA Intern. Med.* **2015**, *175*, 363–371. [CrossRef] [PubMed]
26. Curtis, J.R.; Vincent, J.L. Ethics and end-of-life care for adults in the intensive care unit. *Lancet* **2010**, *376*, 1347–1353. [CrossRef] [PubMed]
27. Kompanje, E.J.O. Burnout, boreout and compassion fatigue on the ICU: It is not about work stress, but about lack of existential significance and professional performance. *Intensive Care Med.* **2018**, *44*, 690–691. [CrossRef] [PubMed]
28. Bolosi, M.; Peritogiannis, V.; Tzimas, P.; Margaritis, A.; Milios, K.; Rizos, D.V. Depressive and Anxiety Symptoms in Relatives of Intensive Care Unit Patients and the Perceived Need for Support. *J. Neurosci. Rural. Pract.* **2018**, *9*, 522–528. [CrossRef]
29. Rose, L.; Muttalib, F.; Adhikari, N.K.J. Psychological Consequences of Admission to the ICU: Helping Patients and Families. *Jama* **2019**, *322*, 213–215. [CrossRef] [PubMed]
30. Jezierska, N. Psychological reactions in family members of patients hospitalised in intensive care units. *Anaesthesiol. Intensive Ther.* **2014**, *46*, 42–45. [CrossRef] [PubMed]
31. Kourti, M.; Christofilou, E.; Kallergis, G. Anxiety and depression symptoms in family members of ICU patients. *Av. Enfermería* **2015**, *33*, 47–54. [CrossRef]
32. Wong, P.; Liamputtong, P.; Koch, S.; Rawson, H. Searching for meaning: A grounded theory of family resilience in adult ICU. *J. Clin. Nurs.* **2019**, *28*, 781–791. [CrossRef]
33. Rawal, G.; Yadav, S.; Kumar, R. Post-intensive Care Syndrome: An Overview. *J. Transl. Int. Med.* **2017**, *5*, 90–92. [CrossRef]
34. Lind, R.; Lorem, G.F.; Nortvedt, P.; Hevrøy, O. Family members' experiences of "wait and see" as a communication strategy in end-of-life decisions. *Intensive Care Med.* **2011**, *37*, 1143–1150. [CrossRef]
35. Thompson, B.T.; Cox, P.N.; Antonelli, M.; Carlet, J.M.; Cassell, J.; Hill, N.S.; Hinds, C.J.; Pimentel, J.M.; Reinhart, K.; Thijs, L.G. Challenges in end-of-life care in the ICU: Statement of the 5th International Consensus Conference in Critical Care: Brussels, Belgium, April 2003: Executive summary. *Crit. Care Med.* **2004**, *32*, 1781–1784. [CrossRef]
36. Shin, K.; Mok, J.H.; Lee, S.H.; Kim, E.J.; Seok, N.R.; Ryu, S.S.; Ha, M.N.; Lee, K. The current status of medical decision-making for dying patients in a medical intensive care unit: A single-center study. *Korean J. Crit. Care Med.* **2014**, *29*, 160–165. [CrossRef]
37. Bailey, J.J.; Sabbagh, M.; Loiselle, C.G.; Boileau, J.; McVey, L. Supporting families in the ICU: A descriptive correlational study of informational support, anxiety, and satisfaction with care. *Intensive Crit. Care Nurs.* **2010**, *26*, 114–122. [CrossRef] [PubMed]
38. Hinkle, J.L.; Fitzpatrick, E. Needs of American relatives of intensive care patients: Perceptions of relatives, physicians and nurses. *Intensive Crit. Care Nurs.* **2011**, *27*, 218–225. [CrossRef] [PubMed]
39. Alvarez, G.F.; Kirby, A.S. The perspective of families of the critically ill patient: Their needs. *Curr. Opin. Crit Care* **2006**, *12*, 614–618. [CrossRef] [PubMed]
40. Bijttebier, P.; Vanoost, S.; Delva, D.; Ferdinande, P.; Frans, E. Needs of relatives of critical care patients: Perceptions of relatives, physicians and nurses. *Intensive Care Med.* **2001**, *27*, 160–165. [CrossRef]
41. Youngner, S.J. Who defines futility? *Jama* **1988**, *260*, 2094–2095. [CrossRef]
42. Schneiderman, L.J.; Jecker, N.S.; Jonsen, A.R. Medical futility: Its meaning and ethical implications. *Ann. Intern. Med.* **1990**, *112*, 949–954. [CrossRef]
43. Wilkinson, D.J.; Savulescu, J. Knowing when to stop: Futility in the ICU. *Curr. Opin. Anaesthesiol.* **2011**, *24*, 160–165. [CrossRef]
44. Keenan, A.; Joseph, L. The needs of family members of severe traumatic brain injured patients during critical and acute care: A qualitative study. *Can. J. Neurosci. Nurs.* **2010**, *32*, 25–35. [PubMed]
45. Huynh, T.N.; Kleerup, E.C.; Raj, P.P.; Wenger, N.S. The opportunity cost of futile treatment in the ICU*. *Crit. Care Med.* **2014**, *42*, 1977–1982. [CrossRef] [PubMed]
46. Mathews, K.S.; Durst, M.S.; Vargas-Torres, C.; Olson, A.D.; Mazumdar, M.; Richardson, L.D. Effect of Emergency Department and ICU Occupancy on Admission Decisions and *Outcomes* for Critically Ill Patients. *Crit. Care Med.* **2018**, *46*, 720–727. [CrossRef]
47. McKiernan, M.; McCarthy, G. Family members' lived experience in the intensive care unit: A phemenological study. *Intensive Crit. Care Nurs.* **2010**, *26*, 254–261. [CrossRef] [PubMed]
48. Schenker, Y.; Crowley-Matoka, M.; Dohan, D.; Tiver, G.A.; Arnold, R.M.; White, D.B. I don't want to be the one saying 'we should just let him die': Intrapersonal tensions experienced by surrogate decision makers in the ICU. *J. Gen. Intern. Med.* **2012**, *27*, 1657–1665. [CrossRef]

Disclaimer/Publisher's Note: The statements, opinions and data contained in all publications are solely those of the individual author(s) and contributor(s) and not of MDPI and/or the editor(s). MDPI and/or the editor(s) disclaim responsibility for any injury to people or property resulting from any ideas, methods, instructions or products referred to in the content.

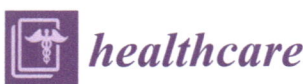 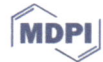

Article

Competency in ECG Interpretation and Arrhythmias Management among Critical Care Nurses in Saudi Arabia: A Cross Sectional Study

Mohammed Saeed Aljohani

Medical-Surgical Nursing Department, Nursing College, Taibah University, Al-Madinah 42362, Saudi Arabia; msejohani@taibahu.edu.sa

Abstract: Background: Electrographic interpretation skills are important for healthcare practitioners caring for patients in need of cardiac assessment. Competency in ECG interpretation skills is critical to determine any abnormalities and initiate the appropriate care required. The purpose of the study was to determine the level of competence in electrocardiographic interpretation and knowledge in arrhythmia management of nurses in critical care settings. Methods: A descriptive cross-sectional design was used. A convenience sample of 255 critical care nurses from 4 hospitals in the Al-Madinah Region in Saudi Arabia was used. A questionnaire was designed containing a participant's characteristics and 10 questions with electrocardiographic strips. A pilot test was carried out to evaluate the validity and reliability of the questionnaire. Descriptive and bivariate analyses were conducted using an independent t-test, one-way ANOVA, or bi-variate correlation tests, as appropriate. A statistical significance of $p < 0.05$ was assumed. Results: Females comprised 87.5% of the sample, and the mean age of the sample was 32.1 (SD = 5.37) years. The majority of the participants (94.9%) had taken electrocardiographic interpretation training courses. The mean total score of correct answers of all 10 ECG strips was 6.45 (±2.54) for ECG interpretation and 4.76 (±2.52) for arrhythmia management. No significant differences were observed between ECG competency level and nursing experience or previous training. Nurses working in the ICU and CCU scored significantly higher than those working in ED. Conclusions: The electrocardiographic knowledge in ECG interpretation and arrhythmia management of critical care nurses is low. Therefore, improving critical care nurses' knowledge of ECGs, identification, and management of cardiac arrhythmias is essential.

Keywords: electrocardiography; interpretation; critical care nursing; competency

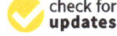

Citation: Aljohani, M.S. Competency in ECG Interpretation and Arrhythmias Management among Critical Care Nurses in Saudi Arabia: A Cross Sectional Study. *Healthcare* **2022**, *10*, 2576. https://doi.org/10.3390/healthcare10122576

Academic Editor: Christina Alexopoulou

Received: 13 November 2022
Accepted: 16 December 2022
Published: 19 December 2022

Publisher's Note: MDPI stays neutral with regard to jurisdictional claims in published maps and institutional affiliations.

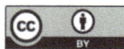

Copyright: © 2022 by the author. Licensee MDPI, Basel, Switzerland. This article is an open access article distributed under the terms and conditions of the Creative Commons Attribution (CC BY) license (https://creativecommons.org/licenses/by/4.0/).

1. Introduction

The prevalence of cardiac arrhythmias, electrical heart conduction system diseases, and other cardiovascular diseases (CVD), in general, is increasing worldwide [1–3]. Cardiac arrhythmias are defined as a disturbance in the normal heart electrical conduction system, resulting in ineffective cardiac pumping, unstable hemodynamic, or cardiac arrest events [2]. Cardiac arrhythmia is one of the leading causes of death globally. In 2016, the World Health Organization (WHO) estimated that 31% (17.9 million) of all global deaths were caused by CVDs [4]. In Saudi Arabia, the WHO and the Ministry of Health (MOH) Statistical Yearbook revealed that cardiovascular diseases were responsible for 42% of non-communicable disease deaths in 2010 [5].

Electrocardiogram (ECG) is a valuable non-invasive diagnostic tool for rapid identification of many heart diseases, especially electrico-cardiac arrhythmias and acute coronary syndrome [6–8]. ECG monitoring is commonly indicated for patients who have a risk of arrhythmias or suspected ischemic heart disease [9,10]. Nurses play a critical role in providing care in critical care settings such as the emergency department (ED), intensive care unit (ICU), and cardiac care unit (CCU) [11,12]. Usually, patients in these departments require ECG monitoring.

Thus, they are required to have sufficient knowledge and skills to provide comprehensive and safe healthcare for all patients with different cardiac diseases, particularly the critically ill in hospitals [13,14].

Nurses usually are the first clinicians to look at the ECG results and to identify abnormalities in the ECG which may require immediate attention. Therefore, it is vital that nurses are competent to carry out an initial assessment and make an early identification and quick decisions to manage ECG abnormalities and activate appropriate emergency health teams or initiate first-line treatments [15–17]. Nurses' rapid and accurate interpretation of cardiac arrhythmias has been linked to safe practices and positive patient outcomes [18–22].

No consensus exists in the literature about the meaning of competency in ECG interpretation and the cut-off point for competency. However, it has been stated that competency can be defined as the ability to have sound understanding of the theoretical and procedural knowledge to interpret cardiac rhythms (knowledge), the ability to recognize cardiac rhythms (skills), and possession of a reasonable level of confidence to effectively undertake the task (attitude) [19].

Several studies conducted worldwide have reported different levels of nurse competency in arrhythmia interpretation and management [10,23–28]. For example, one study reported low competency in ECG interpretation among emergency nurses [29]. In a Turkish study, a high proportion (61%) of bedside nurses reported they did not know the correct practice for ECG monitoring or the correct interpretation of arrhythmias [24]. Another study, conducted in Iraq to investigate nurses' knowledge of early interventional treatment for patients with ventricular tachycardia, showed nurses lack knowledge of how to interpret an ECG and recognize ventricular tachycardia arrhythmias [27]. However, other studies reported high competency scores in ECG interpretation. For example, a 2017 study reported ECG knowledge was high among ED nurses [23]. They also found that knowledge was influenced by ECG training in the previous five years but was not influenced by work experience or the hospital type.

In relation to nurses' knowledge about early intervention for arrhythmia, two previous studies reported a low level of nurses' knowledge regarding management of life-threatening ventricular arrhythmias [26,27]. However, there is a scarcity of studies in Saudi Arabia evaluating nurses' competency in the interpretation of ECG. In fact, only one study was published in this area in 2022 [30]. That study sought to identify nurses' competencies in ECG interpretation. The study focused on their ability to identify cardiac arrhythmia; however, it did not investigate knowledge of proper/initial management.

Therefore, this study aims to identify the level of competency in ECG interpretation, including the ability to identify arrhythmia and its initial management among nurses working in critical care settings in the Al-Madinah region, Saudi Arabia. It is expected that the findings of this study will be beneficial to understand the current nurses' competency in ECG interpretation and arrhythmias management. Furthermore, it is expected to help in establishing nursing programs that enhance nurses' knowledge and skills in relation to ECG interpretation and arrhythmias management.

Study Objectives

Specific objectives of this study were to identify: (1) critical care nurses' competency levels in ECG interpretation and arrhythmia management, (2) relationship between critical care nurses' ECG interpretation and arrhythmia management, and (3) the relationship between participants' demographic and work data and competency level in ECG interpretation and arrhythmia management.

2. Materials and Methods

2.1. Study Design

A descriptive cross-sectional design was used to determine critical care nurses' knowledge about common cardiac arrhythmia interpretation and management.

2.2. Sample and Settings

A convenience sampling method was used to recruit critical care nurses working in critical care units at four main governmental hospitals in two large cities in the Al-Madinah region in Saudi Arabia. These four central hospitals provide a wide range of care for patients with different medical disorders, including cardiac diseases.

To address the objectives of this study, nurses from the selected hospitals who, at the time of data collection, were working in critical care settings including the intensive care unit (ICU), coronary care unit (CCU), and emergency department (ED) were invited to participate. Excluded were nurses who do not provide direct care or are not currently working in critical care units.

The estimated sample size was calculated using G* power software [31]. The effective sample size was determined according to the type of analysis (correlation and Chi square analysis), a medium effect size of (0.3), the power analysis level of (0.80), and a significant p value of (0.05). Based on previous data, the minimal effective sample size was calculated to range between 158 (for correlation analysis) and 221 nurses (for Chi square analysis). A total of 270 questionnaires were returned, and 15 questionnaires were excluded for being incomplete; 255 completed questionnaires were collected and used for the final analysis of this study.

2.3. Procedure

The researcher visited the selected hospitals to recruit study participants. The researcher approached head nurses of the critical care units in each hospital to explain the purpose of this study and to disseminate the link to the online questionnaire, through email or WhatsApp, to the participants. The online questionnaire included an explanation of the objectives of the study and provided instructions on how to complete the questionnaire that was used for data collection. Printed versions of the questionnaire were also provided to the head nurses to promote participation and to increase the response rate. The online survey was hosted on a special webpage created expressly for this purpose. All replies were made to this webpage then extracted to a SPSS file for analysis.

2.4. Instrument

The goal of this study was to understand the competence in interpreting an ECG and the knowledge of first line management for selected arrhythmias. A structured questionnaire was developed and utilized for collecting data to address the objectives of this study. The questionnaire consists of two parts. Part 1 elicited demographic data (age, gender, nationality, qualification, hospital, working area experience, electrocardiographic training, and type of training). Part 2 presented 10 lead II ECG strips. The selected ECG strips were all made with the same technique (tracing speed and calibration, ECG voltage, and same paper) to prevent any technical variations or negatively influence the recognition of arrhythmias. For each strip, participants were asked to answer three questions. No. 1: participants were requested to identify (interpret) the displayed rhythm by selecting one answer only out of eleven possible answers. No. 2: participants were asked to rate the difficulty identifying the cardiac arrhythmia on a three-level scale (1 = easy, 2 = moderate, 3 = difficult). No. 3: participants were asked to identify the initial (first line) management of the cardiac arrhythmia shown in the ECG strip by selecting one answer only out of four possible answers (Table 1). The questions were developed by the author based on reviewing different resources, including textbooks related to ECG interpretation and management of cardiac arrhythmias [32–34], and guidelines of basic life support, cardiopulmonary resuscitation, and advance cardiac life support published by the American Heart Association [35,36].

Table 1. Example of the questionnaire questions.

	For each of the following ECG strips, please select the correct rhythm interpretation and also rate the level of difficulty that was required to interpret each strip on a scale of 1 to 3
Question No 1	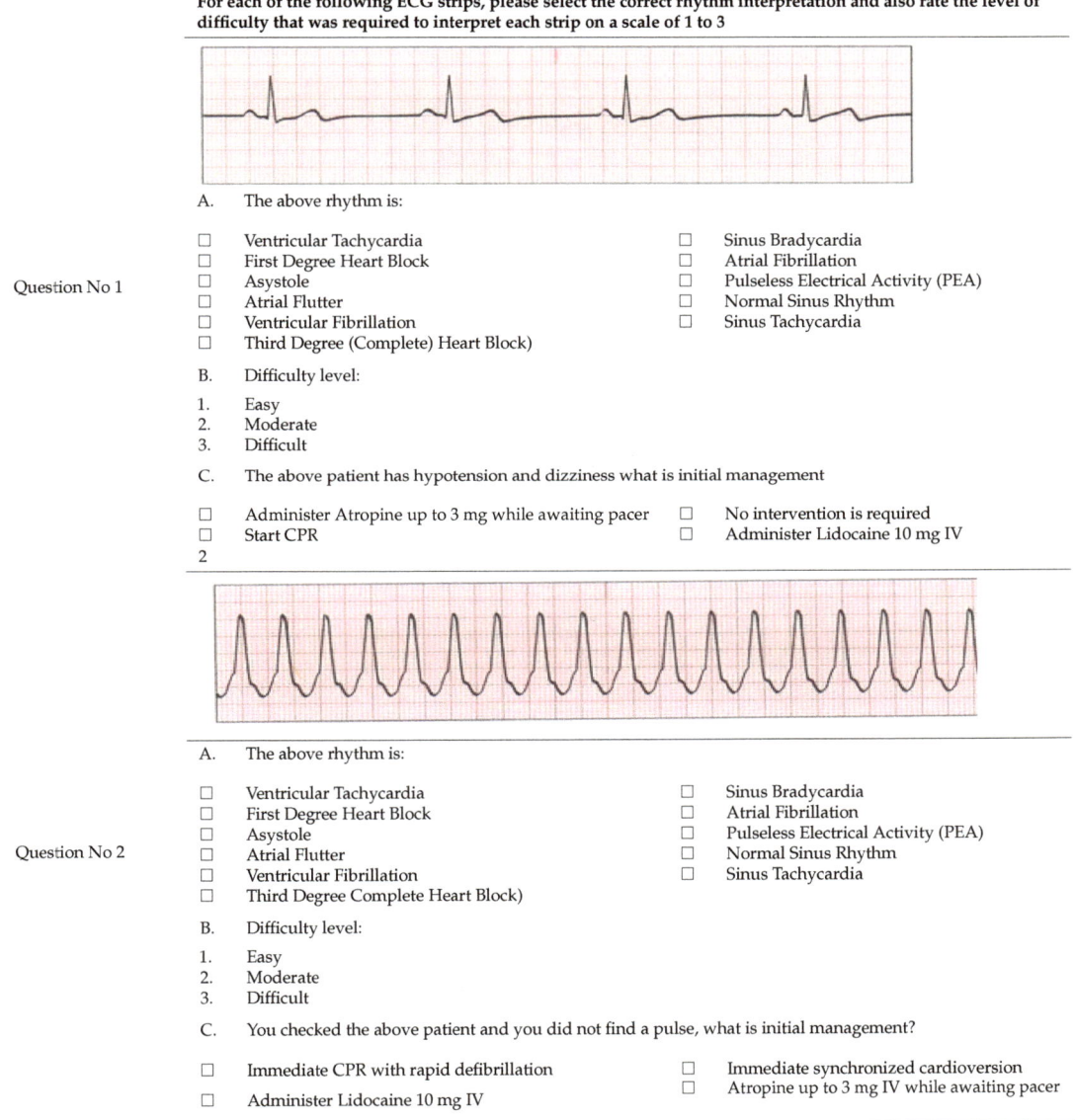 A. The above rhythm is: ☐ Ventricular Tachycardia ☐ Sinus Bradycardia ☐ First Degree Heart Block ☐ Atrial Fibrillation ☐ Asystole ☐ Pulseless Electrical Activity (PEA) ☐ Atrial Flutter ☐ Normal Sinus Rhythm ☐ Ventricular Fibrillation ☐ Sinus Tachycardia ☐ Third Degree (Complete) Heart Block B. Difficulty level: 1. Easy 2. Moderate 3. Difficult C. The above patient has hypotension and dizziness what is initial management ☐ Administer Atropine up to 3 mg while awaiting pacer ☐ No intervention is required ☐ Start CPR ☐ Administer Lidocaine 10 mg IV 2
Question No 2	A. The above rhythm is: ☐ Ventricular Tachycardia ☐ Sinus Bradycardia ☐ First Degree Heart Block ☐ Atrial Fibrillation ☐ Asystole ☐ Pulseless Electrical Activity (PEA) ☐ Atrial Flutter ☐ Normal Sinus Rhythm ☐ Ventricular Fibrillation ☐ Sinus Tachycardia ☐ Third Degree Complete Heart Block) B. Difficulty level: 1. Easy 2. Moderate 3. Difficult C. You checked the above patient and you did not find a pulse, what is initial management? ☐ Immediate CPR with rapid defibrillation ☐ Immediate synchronized cardioversion ☐ Administer Lidocaine 10 mg IV ☐ Atropine up to 3 mg IV while awaiting pacer

The maximum score for interpretation and management questions was 10 points, with each corrected question given 1 point. Participants who scored at least 7.5 out of 10 points were deemed competent in electrocardiographic interpretation and/or management of patients with types of CVD [23]. Conversely, those who scored less than 7.5 points were not considered competent.

To assess the clarity, readability, and reliability of the developed questionnaire, a pilot study was conducted by recruiting 20 nurses from 2 hospitals not included in the final study. Minor revisions were made based on written feedback received from the piloted nurses. The internal reliability of the developed questionnaire was good (Cronbach's alpha = 0.85). Two PhD holders in critical nursing and two ICU consultants, who are experts in clinical health research and cardiac arrhythmia interpretations and management, reviewed the questionnaire to assess the validity, clarity, and feasibility of the developed questionnaire. Some modifications were made to the tool based on expert suggestions.

2.5. Ethical Considerations

Institutional Review Board approval was obtained from the General Directorate of Health Affairs in Madinah (H-03-M-084) before the commencement of this study. Participants were informed that participation is voluntary, names are not required, and they can withdraw from the study at any time. Informed consent was assumed if participants returned a completed questionnaire. Data were confidential; no one, except the investigator, had the authority to view the data. No names were sought; instead, an ID number was assigned to each questionnaire.

2.6. Data Analysis

Statistical Package of Social Science (SPSS) software program (version 22) was used to analyze the data. Descriptive statistics were used to describe participants' characteristics. Chi square tests were utilized to identify the relationship between those who correctly interpreted the ECG strips and correctly identified the management of cardiac arrhythmia in each ECG strip. Independent sample t-test, one way ANOVA, and bi-variate correlation tests were conducted, as appropriate, to determine the association between demographical and work data, participants' knowledge about ECG arrhythmia interpretation, and management. A p value of less than 0.05 was considered a significant value.

3. Results

3.1. The Participants' Sociodemographic

The majority of participants were female (87.5%, n = 223) and non-Saudi citizens (63.9%, n = 163). The mean age of participants was 32.1 years (SD = 5.37). Two-thirds of nurses (75.7%, n = 193) had Bachelor's degrees and three years or less of experience (44.7%). More than half of the participants were working at ICUs (59.2%, n = 151). Most had taken training courses related to cardiac rhythm interpretation or arrhythmia management (94.9%), and 63.9% had completed at minimum the basic life support (BLS) course (Table 2).

Table 2. Sociodemographic of the study population.

Variable	n	%
Gender		
Male	32	12.5%
Female	223	87.5%
Nationality		
Saudi	92	36.1%
Non-Saudi	163	63.9%
Educational qualification		
Nursing Diploma	53	20.8%
Bachelor	193	75.7%
Postgraduate (Diploma, Master, or PhD)	9	3.5%
Current working area		
Intensive care unit (ICU)	151	59.2%
Coronary care unit (CCU)	38	14.9%
Emergency department	66	25.9%
Working experience in the current area		
Less than one year	29	11.4%
1 to 3 years	85	33.3%
4 to 6 years	46	18.0%
7 to 10 years	46	18.0%
More than 10 years	49	19.2%

Table 2. Cont.

Variable	n	%
Did you attend any training in cardiac rhythm interpretation or arrhythmia management?		
Yes	242	94.9%
No	13	5.1%
What type of training attended? *		
ECG interpretation	133	52.1%
Basic life support (BLS)	163	63.9%
Advance cardiac life support	124	48.6%
	Mean (±SD)	Median	Min.–Max.
Age (years)	32.1 (±5.37)	30	23–52

* The participants attended more than one training program or course.

3.2. Knowledge in ECG Interpretation

Participants' competency on ECG interpretation knowledge was low. As shown in Table 2, the mean total score of correct answers of all 10 ECG strips was 6.45 (±2.54) (out of 10). Only 38 participants (14.9%) recognized all 10 ECG arrhythmias correctly, while almost one-fourth (27.1%) of participants answered 8 or more questions correctly, and 45.5% of participants scored 6 correct answers or less. The most frequently identified items (94.1% and 75.7%, respectively) were ECG strip No. 5 (asystole) and ECG strip No. 2 (ventricular tachycardia). Additionally, about two-thirds of participants were correctly able to identify the interpretation of ECG strip No. 7 (sinus tachycardia) (65.1%), and ECG strip No. 10, pulseless electrical activity (PEA) (63.1%). Moreover, about half of the participants were correctly able to identify the interpretation of ECG strip No. 3, ventricular fibrillation (53.7%), ECG strip No. 4, atrial flutter (58.4%), ECG strip No. 8, atrial fibrillation (50.2%), and ECG strip No. 9, third degree complete heart block (56.9%). Almost 30% of participants failed to identify a normal sinus rhythm.

Furthermore, participants were asked about the difficulty in identifying the ECG rhythm based on three levels (1 = easy, 2 = moderate, 3 = difficult). The majority (64.9%) perceived the interpretation of the provided ECG cases as easy, the total mean score was 1.7 (±0.5). Of all participants, 81.2% said ECG strip No. 5 (asystole) was easy to interpret. Moreover, 30.2% said ECG strip No. 3 (ventricular fibrillation) was difficult to interpret (Table 3).

Table 3. Distribution by percentage of nurses' ECG interpretation results.

Participants' Interpretation of ECG Strips	Correct Answer	Participants' Response	
		Correct n (%)	Incorrect n (%)
Interpretation of ECG 1	sinus bradycardia	173 (67.8%)	82 (32.2%)
Interpretation of ECG 2	ventricular tachycardia	193 (75.7%)	62 (24.3%)
Interpretation of ECG 3	ventricular fibrillation	137 (53.7%)	118 (46.3%)
Interpretation of ECG 4	atrial flutter	149 (58.4%)	106 (41.6%)
Interpretation of ECG 5	asystole	240 (94.1%)	15 (5.9%)
Interpretation of ECG 6	normal sinus rhythm	177 (69.4%)	78 (30.6%)
Interpretation of ECG 7	sinus tachycardia	166 (65.1%)	89 (34.9%)
Interpretation of ECG 8	atrial fibrillation	128 (50.2%)	127 (49.8%)
Interpretation of ECG 9	third degree complete heart block	145 (56.9%)	110 (43.1%)
Interpretation of ECG 10	pulseless electrical activity	161 (63.1%)	94 (36.9%)

Table 3. Cont.

Participants' Interpretation of ECG Strips	Correct Answer		Participants' Response	
			Correct *n* (%)	Incorrect *n* (%)
	Mean (±SD)	Median	Minimum–maximum	
Total score of correct interpretation of all 10 ECG strips	6.45 (±2.54)	7.0	1–10	
Total mean score of perceived difficulties in interpretation of all 10 ECG strips	1.70 (±0.51)	1.7	1–3	

3.3. Knowledge of Arrhythmia Management

Participants' competency on first line management of ECG arrhythmias was low. The mean total score of correct answers of all 10 ECGs was 4.76 (±2.52) (out of 10). No one correctly identified all 10 ECG arrhythmias, while 61.6% of participants identified 6 correct answers or less. The most frequently known and correctly identified management (79.6%) was ECG strip No. 5 (asystole). As seen in Table 4, only 32.9% identified the correct first line management for ECG strip No. 8 (atrial fibrillation).

Table 4. Nurses' arrhythmia management results by percentage.

ECG Strip Number (Patient's Condition)	Correct Answer	Participants' Response	
		Correct *n* (%)	Incorrect *n* (%)
ECG 1: Sinus Bradycardia (The patient has hypotension and dizziness)	Administer atropine up to 3 mg while awaiting pacer	117 (45.9%)	138 (54.1%)
ECG 2: Ventricular Tachycardia (You checked the above patient and did not find a pulse)	Immediate CPR with rapid defibrillation	141 (55.3%)	114 (44.7%)
ECG 3: Ventricular Fibrillation	Immediate CPR with rapid defibrillation	125 (49%)	130 (51%)
ECG 4: Atrial Flutter (This patient is hemodynamically unstable)	Synchronized electrical cardioversion	138 (54.1%)	117 (45.9%)
ECG 5: Asystole	Immediate CPR and epinephrine 1 mg IV bolus every 3–5 min	203 (79.6%)	52 (20.4%)
ECG 6: Normal Sinus Rhythm	No intervention required	160 (62.7%)	95 (37.3%)
ECG 7: Sinus Tachycardia (This patient has a pulse but is hemodynamically unstable)	Perform immediate synchronized cardioversion	142 (55.7%)	113 (44.3%)
ECG 8: Atrial Fibrillation (This patient is hemodynamical unstable)	Perform immediate synchronized cardioversion	84 (32.9%)	171 (67.1%)
ECG 9: Complete Third-Degree Heart Block	Administer atropine and perform temporary pacemaker	118 (46.3%)	137 (53.7%)
ECG 10: Pulseless Electrical Activity (PEA)	CPR along with epinephrine	127 (49.8%)	128 (50.2%)
	Mean (±SD)	Median	Minimum-maximum
Total score of correct management of all 10 ECG strips	4.76 (±2.52)	5.0	1–10

As shown in Table 5, Chi square tests show significant relationships between correct interpretation of all ECG strips and correctly identifying the management for each ECG strip. In other words, participants who were more knowledgeable about interpretation of ECG strips were more knowledgeable about the management of cardiac arrhythmias (Table 4).

Table 5. Relationship between participants' ECG interpretation knowledge and arrhythmias management.

ECG Strip No.	Total Correct Management	Incorrect ECG Interpretation and Correct Management	Correct ECG Interpretation and Correct Management	Chi Square (X2)	p Value
ECG 1	137 (53.7%)	20 (14.6%)	117 (85.4%)	41.8	<0.001
ECG 2	174 (68.2%)	33 (19.0%)	141 (81.0%)	8.5	0.005
ECG 3	204 (80.0%)	79 (38.7%)	125 (61.3%)	23.4	<0.001
ECG 4	221 (86.7%)	83 (37.6%)	138 (62.4%)	10.98	0.001
ECG 5	210 (82.4%)	7 (3.3%)	203 (96.7%)	13.97	0.001
ECG 6	180 (70.6%)	20 (11.1%)	160 (88.9%)	109.35	<0.001
ECG 7	166 (65.1%)	24 (14.5%)	142 (85.5%)	171.8	<0.001
ECG 8	138 (54.1%)	54 (39.1%)	84 (60.9%)	13.71	<0.001
ECG 9	184 (72.2%)	66 (35.9%)	118 (64.1%)	14.23	<0.001
ECG 10	139 (54.5%)	12 (8.6%)	127 (91.4%)	104.62	<0.001

3.4. Factors Associated with ECG Interpretation and Arrhythmias Management Knowledge

Several variables were examined for an association between ECG interpretation and the knowledge of arrhythmias management score. Using the independent samples t-test, the nationality (Saudi and non-Saudi) was found to have a significant effect on the ECG interpretation and arrhythmias management knowledge score ($t(253) = 2.022$, $p = 0.044$) for interpretation and ($t(253) = 2.978$, $p = 0.003$) for management. The mean score for non-Saudi nurses ($M = 6.78$, $SD = 2.51$ and $M = 5.11$, $SD = 2.49$) was slightly higher (Table 5) compared to the Saudi nurses ($M = 6.11$, $SD = 2.53$ and $M = 4.15$, $SD = 2.46$).

Regarding the association between what unit the nurse worked on with the ECG interpretation and arrhythmias management knowledge score, results showed a statistically significant difference between groups as determined by one-way ANOVA ($F(3) = 6.80$, $p = 0.01$ for interpretation, and $F(2) = 12.67$, $p = 0.001$ for management. A Tukey post hoc test revealed the mean score for nurses in the ED ($M = 5.42$ and 3.48) was statistically significantly lower than those working in the ICU ($M = 6.99$, 5.25, $p = 0.01$) and CCU ($M = 6.71$ and 5.07, $p = 0.001$). There was no statistically significant difference between the ICU and CCU mean score ($p = 0.918$).

Additionally, a Pearson correlation coefficient was computed to assess the relationship between the participants' perceived difficulty level and the ECG interpretation and arrhythmias management knowledge. There was a moderate negative correlation between the two variables, $r = -0.58$ and -0.55, $p \leq 0.00$. In other words, participants who rated interpretation of the ECG as difficult were more likely to obtain low scores in both ECG interpretation and arrhythmia management.

Regarding other factors studied, results show there were no statistically significant differences, at the $p < 0.05$ level, between the ECG interpretation and arrhythmias management knowledge scores and age ($p = 0.35$) for interpretation and ($p = 0.23$) for management, gender ($p = 0.85$) for interpretation and ($p = 0.58$) for management, previous training ($p = 0.18$) for interpretation and ($p = 0.25$) for management, qualifications ($p = 0.51$) for interpretation and ($p = 0.21$) management, or work experience ($p = 0.47$) for interpretation and ($p = 0.42$) for management, (Table 6).

Table 6. Correlation between participants' demographic characteristics, knowledge about management of ECG arrhythmias, and participants' knowledge about interpretation of ECG strip scenarios.

Variables	Participants' Knowledge about Interpretation of ECG Rhythm		Participants' Knowledge about Management of Cardiac Arrhythmias	
	Correlation (r)	p Value	Correlation (r)	p Value
Age (years)	0.06	0.35	0.08	0.23
Gender (female)	0.01	0.88	0.04	0.56
Nationality (non-Saudi)	0.12	0.051	0.18	0.004
Educational qualification	0.16	0.01	0.19	0.003
Working experience in the current area	−0.04	0.48	−0.04	0.58
Attendance of training program/ course about cardiac rhythm interpretation or arrhythmia management	0.17	0.03	0.23	0.02
Perceived difficulties in interpretation of all 10 ECG strips (Total score out of 30)	−0.58	<0.001	−0.55	<0.001
Participants' knowledge about management of ECG arrhythmias			0.93	<0.001

4. Discussion

The aim of this study was to identify nurses' competency in ECG interpretation and arrhythmia management in critical care settings in four hospitals in the Al-Madinah region in Saudi Arabia. To the best of my knowledge, this is the first study to evaluate critical care nurses' competency in ECG interpretation and arrythmias management in Saudi Arabia.

The competency level in this study was set at 7.5 out of 10. Results of the study showed overall ECG interpretation among nurses working in critical care settings (ICU, CCU and ED) was below the preset threshold (7.5 out of 10). The mean total score of correct answers of all 10 ECGs was 6.45 (±2.54). This finding is consistent with the results of other local and international studies [29,30,37]. A recent study in Saudi Arabia found that 50% of nurses working in the ICU and CCU showed low competency in ECG interpretations [30]. The total mean score was 6.68 out of 10. However, the competency level in the present study is lower than in other studies [23,38]. When Coll-Badell et al. evaluated the knowledge of nurses in the ED, they found competency was high, where 93% of nurses scored 7.5 or more, with the average score of 8.6 out of 10 [23].

In the current study, only 14.9% of participants answered all 10 questions correctly. This finding is similar to Ho et al., that found 12.5% of participants correctly answered all the questions [38].

The findings of the present study showed the questions that were most often answered correctly were related to asystole (94%) and ventricular tachycardia (75.7%). However, one study, in contrast, found nurses' ability to identify ventricular tachycardia was low (22%) [39]. The majority of participants in this study (81.2%) perceived the interpretation of the ECG involving asystole as easy. Given that most of the nurses in this study had completed BLS (63.9%) or ACLS (48.6%) courses, it is not surprising they can identify the asystole rhythm correctly and know how it should be managed. This finding is congruent with other studies [29,38,40]. In addition, the current study found nurses had difficulties identifying atrial flutter (58.4%), atrial fibrillation (50.2%), and third-degree complete heart block (56.9%). This finding was also similar in other studies [28,30,41]. In contrast, Tahboub and Dal Yılmaz found that 84.6% of nurses were able to identify atrial flutter [42]. In addition, about two-thirds of participants were able to interpret ECG strips related to sinus bradycardia, sinus tachycardia, and PEA. It can be argued that nurses need to recognize the normal ECG first to be able to identify any abnormalities. However, the findings showed that one-third of nurses in the current study had difficulty recognizing normal sinus rhythm. This finding was also reported in 2022, which found that 42% of the nurses failed to identify the normal sinus rhythm [30].

The second objective of the current study was to evaluate the competency level of nurses working in the critical care setting to identify first line management for some common fatal arrythmias. The results showed overall competency was below the required limits. The mean total score of correct first line management was 4.76 (±2.52) out of 10. This finding is similar to the findings of two previous studies which revealed the majority of the nurses had unsatisfactory knowledge concerning early management of life-threatening ventricular arrhythmias [26,27]. In the current study, no participant identified the correct first line management for all 10 ECG arrhythmias, while 61.6% identified 6 correct answers or less. The majority of participants (79.6%) identified first line management for asystole, while more than half had difficulties identifying the correct first line management for pulseless electrical activity, third degree complete heart block, atrial fibrillation, and ventricular fibrillation. In more detail, despite the fact more than 50% of the nurses correctly identified the ECG strips for ventricular fibrillation, atrial flutter, atrial fibrillation, and third-degree heart block, less than two-thirds were able to recognize the proper management of these cardiac arrhythmias. Moreover, between 81% and 85.5% of nurses in this study correctly recognized the management of cardiac arrhythmias for sinus bradycardia, ventricular tachycardia, and sinus tachycardia.

The findings of this study showed that there are significant relationships between participants' knowledge about interpretation of ECG strip scenarios and management of ECG arrhythmias. These expected results indicated that nurses with a strong knowledge of arrhythmia interpretation were more knowledgeable about correct management of the cardiac arrhythmias and more likely to make sound clinical decisions and take quick interventional actions to manage cardiac arrhythmias [43–45]. Moreover, these findings emphasize the importance for improving critical care nurses' knowledge about interpretation of ECG and early identification of cardiac arrhythmias and correct management of cardiac arrhythmias [44–47].

The finding of this study showed a significant association among participants' accurate knowledge about the interpretation of ECG rhythms, participants' knowledge about management of cardiac arrhythmias, and the nurses' nationality. Non-Saudi nurses scored slightly higher than Saudi nurses. Although this finding is difficult to explain, it may be attributed to the fact there were 163 non-Saudi participants in this study and 92 Saudi participants. However, this finding may indicate a lack of knowledge of ECG interpretation and arrhythmias management among Saudi nurses. Therefore, ECG interpretation knowledge and skills must be addressed in Saudi nursing curricula and continuing education programs.

In addition, the current study found an association between ECG interpretation and arrhythmia management knowledge and the department nurses worked in. Mean score of nurses working in the ICU and CCU was significantly higher than those working in the ED. A similar study found CCU experience was associated with better results on ECG interpretation [37]. Another study revealed that nurses working in the CCU had better ECG knowledge than nurses working in the ICU and ED [48]. Contrary to this current research, a 2021 study found that nurses who had ED experience scored significantly higher than those who did not [38].

Several studies reported improved competency in ECG interpretation of fatal arrhythmias after education [9,25,39]. Logically, nurses with training showed higher scores compared to those without training [23,29,48]. It has been argued that knowledge and skills may diminish with time; therefore, refresher courses are required. Nolan and Coll-Badell et al. recommend that nurses take ECG interpretation courses at least every five years [23,49]. However, the findings of this current study are not consistent with previous research. The current study showed the mean score of participants was not affected by whether or not they had training. Although the majority of participants claimed to have training related to arrhythmia, it was not clear when training occurred or how affective it was. This finding draws attention to the need to evaluate arrhythmia training in both nursing curricula and on-the-job courses.

Data from the current study provided no significant difference among participants' gender, age, qualifications, or work experience and their expertise in ECG interpretation. This result is consistent with two studies that found no correlation between age, work experience, and interpretation knowledge and skills [37,50]. In contrast, Keller et al. reported a positive correlation between years of experience and higher scores [40].

4.1. Research Implications and Recommendations for Clinical Practice

This study provides baseline information to improve the evidence about the level of knowledge of critical care nurses regarding ECG interpretation and cardiac arrhythmia management in Saudi Arabia. Moreover, this study will provide helpful information to educators to develop clinical guidelines and education programs to improve critical care nurses' knowledge and competencies for early identification, assessment, and appropriate management of patients with CVDs, particularly cardiac arrhythmias and CAD.

It is essential to improve critical care nurses' knowledge about monitoring ECGs and identifying cardiac arrhythmias. Several strategies are recommended to achieve this. ECG monitors with automated interpretation are highly recommended in critical care settings to facilitate early detection of abnormal ECG strips and diagnosis of cardiac arrhythmias. Most importantly, the curricula of Bachelor of Science in Nursing programs in Saudi Arabia should be reviewed and adjusted to include topics about ECG interpretations and management of cardiac arrhythmias.

4.2. Limitations

Despite the importance of the findings of this study, there were a few limitations. Using a cross-sectional design will not help identify the effect and causal relationship of the lack of knowledge on interpreting ECG and cardiac arrhythmias. Additionally, using convenience sampling will negatively affect the generalization of the findings for all critical care nurses in Saudi Arabia. This study was limited to only 10 ECG rhythms; other important arrythmias can be included in other studies, such as ST elevation or pathological Q waves.

5. Conclusions

This is the first study in Saudi Arabia to evaluate both ECG interpretation and arrhythmia management knowledge for nurses working in critical care settings. The overall results revealed the majority of nurses in this study were below the preset competency limit for ECG interpretation and arrhythmia management. Therefore, improving critical care nurses' knowledge on monitoring ECGs and identification and management of cardiac arrhythmias is essential. Through collaboration between the health system and education institutions, improvements can be achieved through nursing education and in-service training programs and workshops. Contrary to what several studies found related to the role of training in improving nurses' interpretation knowledge, this current study did not find any significant association. This finding should be carefully examined, as it may indicate weaknesses in current nursing curricula and/or in-service training programs. Conducting further longitudinal and experimental research studies is recommended to investigate the effectiveness of health education programs on critical care nurses' ECG interpretation skills and management of cardiac arrhythmias.

Funding: This research received no external funding.

Institutional Review Board Statement: The study was conducted in accordance with the Declaration of Helsinki and approved by the Institutional Review Board of General Directorate of Health Affairs in Madinah, Saudi Arabia (H-03-M-084 date 2 February 2021).

Informed Consent Statement: Informed consent was obtained from all subjects involved in the study.

Data Availability Statement: The data presented in this study are available on reasonable request from the author. The data are not publicly available due to privacy restrictions.

Acknowledgments: The author would like to thank all the nurses and hospitals participated in this research.

Conflicts of Interest: The authors declare no conflict of interest.

References

1. Chow, G.V.; Marine, J.E.; Fleg, J.L. Epidemiology of arrhythmias and conduction disorders in older adults. *Clin. Geriatr. Med.* **2012**, *28*, 539–553. [CrossRef]
2. Kumar, A.; Avishay, D.M.; Jones, C.R.; Shaikh, J.D.; Kaur, R.; Aljadah, M.; Kichloo, A.; Shiwalkar, N.; Keshavamurthy, S. Sudden cardiac death: Epidemiology, pathogenesis and management. *Rev. Cardiovasc. Med.* **2021**, *22*, 147–158. [CrossRef]
3. Townsend, N.; Kazakiewicz, D.; Wright, F.L.; Timmis, A.; Huculeci, R.; Torbica, A.; Gale, C.P.; Achenbach, S.; Weidinger, F.; Vardas, P. Epidemiology of cardiovascular disease in Europe. *Nat. Rev. Cardiol.* **2022**, *19*, 133–143. [CrossRef]
4. Şahin, B.; İlgün, G. Risk factors of deaths related to cardiovascular diseases in World Health Organization (WHO) member countries. *Health Soc. Care Community* **2022**, *30*, 73–80. [CrossRef]
5. Ministry of Health. Cardiovascular Diseases Cause 42% of Non-Communicable Diseases Deaths in the Kingdom. 2013. Available online: https://www.moh.gov.sa/en/Ministry/MediaCenter/News/Pages/News-2013-10-30-002.aspx (accessed on 20 September 2021).
6. Martis, R.J.; Acharya, U.R.; Adeli, H. Current methods in electrocardiogram characterization. *Comput. Biol. Med.* **2014**, *48*, 133–149. [CrossRef]
7. Sattar, Y.; Chhabra, L. *Electrocardiogram*; StatPearls Publishing, 2021. Available online: https://www.ncbi.nlm.nih.gov/books/NBK549803/ (accessed on 15 November 2022).
8. Goldberger, A.L.; Goldberger, Z.D.; Shvilkin, A. *Clinical Electrocardiography: A Simplified Approach E-Book*; Elsevier Health Sciences: Philadelphia, PA, USA, 2017.
9. Funk, M.; Fennie, K.P.; Stephens, K.E.; May, J.L.; Winkler, C.G.; Drew, B.J. Association of implementation of practice standards for electrocardiographic monitoring with nurses' knowledge, quality of care, and patient outcomes. *Circ. Cardiovasc. Qual. Outcomes* **2017**, *10*, 1–10. [CrossRef]
10. Hernandez, J.M.; Glembocki, M.M.; McCoy, M.A. Increasing Nursing Knowledge of ST-Elevated Myocardial Infarction Recognition on 12-Lead Electrocardiograms to Improve Patient Outcomes. *J. Contin. Educ. Nurs.* **2019**, *50*, 475–480. [CrossRef] [PubMed]
11. Ervin, J.N.; Kahn, J.M.; Cohen, T.R.; Weingart, L.R. Teamwork in the intensive care unit. *Am. Psychol.* **2018**, *73*, 468–477. [CrossRef]
12. Scholtz, S.; Nel, E.W.; Poggenpoel, M.; Myburgh, C.P.H. The Culture of Nurses in a Critical Care Unit. *Glob. Qual. Nurs. Res.* **2016**, *3*, 2333393615625996. [CrossRef] [PubMed]
13. Adhikari, N.K.J.; Rubenfeld, G.D. Worldwide demand for critical care. *Curr. Opin. Crit. Care* **2011**, *17*, 620–625. [CrossRef] [PubMed]
14. Tanaka Gutiez, M.; Ramaiah, R. Demand versus supply in intensive care: An ever-growing problem. *Crit. Care* **2014**, *18* (Suppl. 1), P9. [CrossRef]
15. Haugaa, K.H.; Grenne, B.L.; Eek, C.H.; Ersbøll, M.; Valeur, N.; Svendsen, J.H.; Florian, A.; Sjøli, B.; Brunvand, H.; Køber, L.; et al. Strain echocardiography improves risk prediction of ventricular arrhythmias after myocardial infarction. *JACC Cardiovasc. Imaging* **2013**, *6*, 841–850. [CrossRef] [PubMed]
16. Leren, I.S.; Saberniak, J.; Haland, T.F.; Edvardsen, T.; Haugaa, K.H. Combination of ECG and Echocardiography for Identification of Arrhythmic Events in Early ARVC. *JACC Cardiovasc. Imaging* **2017**, *10*, 503–513. [CrossRef]
17. Weber, R.; Stambach, D.; Jaeggi, E. Diagnosis and management of common fetal arrhythmias. *J. Saudi Heart Assoc.* **2011**, *23*, 61–66. [CrossRef] [PubMed]
18. Evenson, L.; Farnsworth, M. Skilled cardiac monitoring at the bedside: An algorithm for success. *Crit. Care Nurse* **2010**, *30*, 14–22. [CrossRef]
19. Hernández-Padilla, J.M.; Granero-Molina, J.; Márquez-Hernández, V.V.; Suthers, F.; López-Entrambasaguas, O.M.; Fernández-Sola, C. Design and validation of a three-instrument toolkit for the assessment of competence in electrocardiogram rhythm recognition. *Eur. J. Cardiovasc. Nurs.* **2017**, *16*, 425–434. [CrossRef]
20. Ornato, J.P.; Peberdy, M.A.; Reid, R.D.; Feeser, V.R.; Dhindsa, H.S. Impact of resuscitation system errors on survival from in-hospital cardiac arrest. *Resuscitation* **2012**, *83*, 63–69. [CrossRef]
21. Perkins, G.D.; Handley, A.J.; Koster, R.W.; Castrén, M.; Smyth, M.A.; Olasveengen, T.; Monsieurs, K.G.; Raffay, V.; Gräsner, J.T.; Wenzel, V.; et al. European Resuscitation Council Guidelines for Resuscitation 2015. Section 2. Adult basic life support and automated external defibrillation. *Resuscitation* **2015**, *95*, 81–99. [CrossRef]
22. Soar, J.; Nolan, J.P.; Böttiger, B.W.; Perkins, G.D.; Lott, C.; Carli, P.; Pellis, T.; Sandroni, C.; Skrifvars, M.B.; Smith, G.B.; et al. European Resuscitation Council Guidelines for Resuscitation 2015. Section 3. Adult advanced life support. *Resuscitation* **2015**, *95*, 100–147. [CrossRef] [PubMed]
23. Coll-Badell, M.; Jiménez-Herrera, M.F.; Llaurado-Serra, M. Emergency Nurse Competence in Electrocardiographic Interpretation in Spain: A Cross-Sectional Study. *J. Emerg. Nurs.* **2017**, *43*, 560–570. [CrossRef] [PubMed]
24. Doğan, H.D.; Melek, M. Determination of the Abilities of Nurses in Diagnosing the ECG Findings About Emergency Heart Diseases and Deciding the Appropriate Treatment Approaches. *Turkish J. Cardiovasc. Nurs.* **2012**, *3*, 60–69. [CrossRef]
25. Goodridge, E.; Furst, C.; Herrick, J.; Song, J.; Tipton, P.H. Accuracy of cardiac rhythm interpretation by medical-surgical nurses: A pilot study. *J. Nurses Prof. Dev.* **2013**, *29*, 35–40. [CrossRef] [PubMed]
26. Khalil, N.; Abd Rahman, H.; Hamouda, E. Critical care nurses' knowledge and practice regarding life-threatening ventricular dysrhythmias. *Clin. Prac.* **2018**, *15*, 747–753. [CrossRef]

27. Mousa, A.M.; Owaid, H.A.; Ahmed, R.S.; Zedaan, H.A.; Shalal, S.H. Nurses' Knowledge Concerning Early Interventions for Patients with Ventricular Tachycardia at Baghdad Teaching Hospitals. *Kufa J. Nurs. Sci.* **2016**, *6*, 1–9.
28. Ruhwanya, D.I.; Tarimo, E.A.M.; Ndile, M. Life threatening arrhythmias: Knowledge and skills among nurses working in critical care settings at muhimbili national hospital, Dar es Salaam, Tanzania. *Tanzan. J. Health Res.* **2018**, *20*. [CrossRef]
29. Rahimpour, M.; Shahbazi, S.; Ghafourifard, M.; Gilani, N.; Breen, C. Electrocardiogram interpretation competency among emergency nurses and emergency medical service (EMS) personnel: A cross-sectional and comparative descriptive study. *Nurs. Open* **2021**, *8*, 1712–1719. [CrossRef]
30. Alkhalaileh, M.; Mohideen, M. Nurses competencies in Electrocardiogram interpretation: A systematic review. *Biosci. Res.* **2022**, *19*, 874–881.
31. Faul, F.; Erdfelder, E.; Lang, A.; Buchner, A. G* Power 3 [Computer Software] 2007. Available online: https://www.psychologie.hhu.de/arbeitsgruppen/allgemeine-psychologie-und-arbeitspsychologie/gpower (accessed on 15 January 2022).
32. Hampton, J.; Hampton, J. *The ECG Made Easy E-Book*; Elsevier: Edinburgh, UK, 2019.
33. Kusumoto, F. *ECG Interpretation: From Pathophysiology to Clinical Application*; Springer: Cham, Switzerland, 2020; pp. 1–355.
34. Reichlin, T.; Abächerli, R.; Twerenbold, R.; Kühne, M.; Schaer, B.; Müller, C.; Sticherling, C.; Osswald, S. Advanced ECG in 2016: Is there more than just a tracing? *Swiss Med. Wkly.* **2016**, *146*, w14303. [CrossRef]
35. Bhanji, F.; Donoghue, A.J.; Wolff, M.S.; Flores, G.E.; Halamek, L.P.; Berman, J.M.; Sinz, E.H.; Cheng, A. Part 14: Education: 2015 American Heart Association guidelines update for cardiopulmonary resuscitation and emergency cardiovascular care. *Circulation* **2015**, *132*, S561–S573. [CrossRef]
36. Cheng, A.; Magid, D.J.; Auerbach, M.; Bhanji, F.; Bigham, B.L.; Blewer, A.L.; Dainty, K.N.; Diederich, E.; Lin, Y.; Leary, M.; et al. Part 6: Resuscitation education science: 2020 american heart association guidelines for cardiopulmonary resuscitation and emergency cardiovascular care. *Circulation* **2020**, *142*, S551–S579. [CrossRef]
37. Werner, K.; Kander, K.; Axelsson, C. Electrocardiogram interpretation skills among ambulance nurses. *Eur. J. Cardiovasc. Nurs.* **2016**, *15*, 262–268. [CrossRef] [PubMed]
38. Ho, J.K.-M.; Yau, C.H.-Y.; Wong, C.-Y.; Tsui, J.S.-S. Capability of emergency nurses for electrocardiogram interpretation. *Int. Emerg. Nurs.* **2021**, *54*, 100953. [CrossRef] [PubMed]
39. Çıkrıkçı Isık, G.; Şafak, T.; Tandoğan, M.; Çevik, Y. Effectiveness of the CRISP Method on the Primary Cardiac Arrhythmia Interpretation Accuracy of Nurses. *J. Contin. Educ. Nurs.* **2020**, *51*, 574–580. [CrossRef] [PubMed]
40. Keller, K.; Eggenberger, T.; Leavitt, M.A.; Sabatino, D. Acute Care Nurses' Arrhythmia Knowledge: Defining Competency. *J. Contin. Educ. Nurs.* **2020**, *51*, 39–45. [CrossRef]
41. Qaddumi, J.; Almahmoud, O.; Alamri, M.; Maniago, J. Competency in Electrocardiogram Interpretation among Registered Nurses in Private and Government Hospitals In Nablus, Palestine. *Majmaah J. Health Sci.* **2019**, *8*, 70. [CrossRef]
42. Tahboub, O.Y.H.; Dal Yılmaz, Ü. Nurses' knowledge and practices of electrocardiogram interpretation. *Int. Cardiovasc. Res. J.* **2019**, *13*, 80–84.
43. Begg, G.; Willan, K.; Tyndall, K.; Pepper, C.; Tayebjee, M. Electrocardiogram interpretation and arrhythmia management: A primary and secondary care survey. *Br. J. Gen. Pract.* **2016**, *66*, e291–e296. [CrossRef]
44. Chen, Y.; Kunst, E.; Nasrawi, D.; Massey, D.; Johnston, A.N.B.; Keller, K.; Fengzhi Lin, F. Nurses' competency in electrocardiogram interpretation in acute care settings: A systematic review. *J. Adv. Nurs.* **2022**, *78*, 1245–1266. [CrossRef]
45. Ebrahim, M.; Alseid, R.; Aleinati, R.; Tuzcu, V. Electrocardiogram interpretation among pediatricians: Assessing knowledge, attitudes, and practice. *Ann. Pediatr. Cardiol.* **2020**, *13*, 205–211. [CrossRef]
46. Alanezi, F. A systematized review aimed to identify the impact of basic electrocardiogram training courses on qualified nurses. *Saudi Crit. Care J.* **2018**, *2*, 51. [CrossRef]
47. Schultz, S.J. Evidence-based strategies for teaching dysrhythmia monitoring practices to staff nurses. *J. Contin. Educ. Nurs.* **2011**, *42*, 308–319. [CrossRef] [PubMed]
48. Zhang, H.; Hsu, L.L. The effectiveness of an education program on nurses' knowledge of electrocardiogram interpretation. *Int. Emerg. Nurs.* **2013**, *21*, 247–251. [CrossRef] [PubMed]
49. Nolan, J.P.; Soar, J.; Zideman, D.A.; Biarent, D.; Bossaert, L.L.; Deakin, C.; Koster, R.W.; Wyllie, J.; Böttiger, B. European Resuscitation Council Guidelines for Resuscitation 2010 Section 1. Executive summary. *Resuscitation* **2010**, *81*, 1219–1276. [CrossRef] [PubMed]
50. Alusaunawy, A. Evaluation of Nurses Knowledge and Practical of Electrocardiogram Toward Adolescent Patient. *IOSR J. Nurs. Health Sci. Ver. II* **2015**, *4*, 10–16. [CrossRef]

MDPI AG
Grosspeteranlage 5
4052 Basel
Switzerland
Tel.: +41 61 683 77 34

Healthcare Editorial Office
E-mail: healthcare@mdpi.com
www.mdpi.com/journal/healthcare

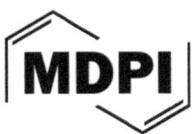

Disclaimer/Publisher's Note: The title and front matter of this reprint are at the discretion of the Guest Editor. The publisher is not responsible for their content or any associated concerns. The statements, opinions and data contained in all individual articles are solely those of the individual Editor and contributors and not of MDPI. MDPI disclaims responsibility for any injury to people or property resulting from any ideas, methods, instructions or products referred to in the content.

www.ingramcontent.com/pod-product-compliance
Lightning Source LLC
LaVergne TN
LVHW070000100526
838202LV00019B/2593